How to Make Wild, Passionate Love to your Man

Jacqueline George

with Eric George

PUBLISHER

Q~Press Publishing

Contents

Foreplay

The shifting battlefield that is sex between men and women is a huge subject. It lies right at the heart of our existence, drives most of our life choices, colours our dreams and is the well from which artists draw endless inspiration. Without sex most works of fiction would be meaningless and poets would be unemployed. Artists and photographers would be limited to landscapes and sunsets.

Immense amounts of instructional material are available on every aspect of lovemaking, and you can find books on anything, from flowers in sex to tying up your lover and tormenting him. You can be forgiven for thinking that there are already more than enough words on paper and no more are needed. So when my editor Jean Marie Stine suggested I write about how to make love to your man, I felt inadequate. The task of telling other women anything about sex was frightening. Sitting at my word processor and sketching out a potential book made me feel very humble.

That must have lasted all of five minutes. Then I became excited at the chance of unbuttoning a few secrets, and letting you peep into the sexy world between your man's ears. It might surprise you; it might frustrate you, but you can trust the ultimate truth of what you read here. And the more you know about how your man views lovemaking, the better you can be at doing it. A good lover not only enjoys herself more, but she is cherished and valued by her man.

Of course, anyone who is insensitive enough to lecture women on being more feminine lays herself open to charges of anti-feminism, a crime worse than High Treason. So let me put my hand on my heart and say that I am an ardent feminist. Not only am I a woman myself but I am quite happy to see us running more and more of our world. Like most women, I respect men and enjoy their company. At the same time, I understand that they like looking at pictures of us posing provocatively nude. This apparent conflict is the theme behind my book; the fact that men cannot separate their love of you from their hunger for your body and the wonderful things you can do with it. I resent the crazy Feminist Front telling me that men can love women but only if they don't think of us as sex objects. Are they mad?

Women were designed to make men think of them as sex objects. If they see a twinkle in your eye, the sway of your hair or your plump, female butt swinging as you walk, what are they meant to think of? Higher math? International economic growth since 1950? Not a hope. They will be thinking of you and sex, and so this book is dedicated to both. I hope you enjoy it.

A quick word and I'm done. All English language writers on sex run up against the problem of how to refer to the human genitalia. This isn't a medical book so I'm not going to use penis and vulva (who can use a word like vulva romantically?). On the other hand the traditional Anglo-Saxon alternatives are so often used as swear words that they don't sit happily next to 'higher thoughts'. Coy expressions like 'her sex' or even worse 'her flower' make me wince. So I have chosen pussy (which at least has the respectability of being more or less the same in French and is therefore cultured), and cock (which isn't cultured at all but doesn't grate on the ear). I hope they are comfortable for you too. If not, they will be by the end of the book because the two of them play the leading roles.

Enough pontificating. Read on and I hope you find the book stimulating and at least a little uncomfortable. If it's useful, congratulate my editor. If it leaves you in a smouldering fury, write to me. As I sit here next to the tropical Coral Sea, coconut palms waving above me, I promise I'll read your complaints and feel very sorry. Honest!

Jacqueline George, May 2005
www.jacquelinegeorgewriter.com

- 1 -

Pussy rules the world.
Madonna

Of course I don't mind him staring after pretty girls.
He's like a dog chasing cars; if he caught one he
wouldn't know what to do with it.
Anon

Excuse me, You have a Problem

So you've caught one, or you have a slightly used one at home. Not a pretty girl of course, but a living, breathing man. The question is, what do you do with him? You want to make wonderful love to him, something he'll never forget, but are you qualified? Your education and experience has not prepared you for this. There were no school courses on lovemaking, although you did learn how to fit a condom and avoid babies and other diseases. Your friends probably know no more about it than you do. You definitely refuse to consult your brother. No good turning to Mother; it would be hard to guess who would be more embarrassed. And besides, watching her with Dad, you have to believe there must be better tutors. So what do you do?

Well, the good news is that lovemaking, like cooking, can be learned. You know very well that with practice and determination you could learn to make a chocolate cake that even your Grandmother would envy. In just the same way you can be confident that practice and determination will bring your lovemaking up to the sophistication of the great courtesans of history. The ones that could enchant a Napoleon and determine the fate of nations with a wiggle of their hips.

Well – let's not exaggerate. You can learn technique in the same way that you can learn bookkeeping, and every lover needs to have some understanding of technique. But what will turn you from a technically competent lover into a great lover is the artistry and imagination you bring with you. Add a little flair and you will become the best lover in town, maybe even the best in your whole state. And you never know – you might have it in you to decide the fate of nations as well. Monica Lewinsky nearly did it, even if her lovemaking proved to be – shall we say – specialized.

What is Lovemaking?

Lovemaking is the sexual interaction of two people leading towards orgasm. It's as simple as that, but that's a very broad definition, in the same way that 'eating food' can cover anything from grabbing a sandwich-to-go at the gas station to the candle-lit dinner in an expensive restaurant with the person you love.

In fact the comparison with eating is a good one. We do both in response to basic physical demands of our bodies. When we are hungry for food or hungry for sex, we dream about it, taste in it our minds. When we finally get to satisfy our hunger, we indulge ourselves until we are satisfied and then feel comfortable and relaxed – until the next time.

Of course, there are differences. Whole cultures have been built up around eating; chefs study for years and are paid handsomely for presenting sophisticated dishes to discerning diners. In contrast, far too many people are stuck at the grab-a-sandwich stage when it comes to sex. They just do what comes naturally often enough to satisfy their hunger and do not aspire to anything more. But that is not what you are looking for. You want the full silver service, soup to cognac and cheese experience.

What do you need to know?

You need to know and understand lots of things if you want to offer your man the superlative lovemaking you are capable of. Perhaps not an armful of college text books, but a lot all the same. However, the good news is that we are not talking about Ancient Greek or Astrophysics. Learning about lovemaking is fun. If any college scheduled it, lovemaking would be the one course that everyone could relate to. It would be constantly over-subscribed and no one would ever drop out.

You need to understand men, look at yourself through their eyes and see what they see. You will try to feel as they feel and anticipate what turns them on (or off). You need to understand yourself, your own sexual requirements and how your hunger is best satisfied. You will learn to orchestrate your lovemaking so that you are teasing, enticing and provoking your man for perhaps hours before he tears your clothes off with his teeth.

And of course you will need some ideas on what to do once he has got you into a horizontal position.

- 2 -

I prefer the simple things in life. Like men.
Anon

*Being a woman is a terribly difficult task since it
consists principally of dealing with men.*
Joseph Conrad

Man – a Solitary Animal?

There is a real question as to whether men actually need women. It is true that they like female company sometimes, but was there a time in their evolutionary past when they behaved just like wandering tomcats? Did they roam from female to female, visiting their nests for tea and sympathy, and of course a little sex if there was any on offer? Left to themselves a large proportion of men would be content to live that way even today. You can probably think of some, unattached or perhaps divorced, who seem to be happy with no more female contact than a tomcat. Women might be interesting to them, but not as important as football, beer, male friends, fishing.

It is a depressing thought that you might take second place to standing up to his waist in cold water for hour after hour waiting for a small fish to bite.

Women have always had a different agenda. Until recently male support was essential to raise children, and still today sharing the burden with a man makes life a lot easier. Women offered men cooked food, warmth, companionship and sex, and in return expected fidelity and protection. Men are adaptable (and possibly lazy), the deal seemed fair enough, and the modern nuclear family was born.

Nowadays women live closely with men, they work with them and enjoy a shared culture. It is normal in western societies for a woman to have men working under her, and female CEO's or frontline soldiers excite no surprise. Argue about the details if you will but in the West the goal of social equality is nearly achieved. Does that mean that men have finally been domesticated? I doubt it. You are still dealing with a different animal, and he thinks in a different way.

Men looking at Women

Dogs might make friends using their noses, but a man's first assessment of a woman will almost certainly be visual. Men are very visual people so if you want to make an impression it helps to look good. The problem is that your idea of what looks good is probably not the same as his.

Every time a man looks at a female, there is an instant evaluation of her sexual potential. In a fraction of a second his brain checks out her age, attractiveness, her clothes and how free she appears to be, and then he will treat her according to the results. Men are very, very quick at this. While walking down the street the females are scanned and the messages come flooding in:

Little old lady. Smile; "Morning!"

Small, nice long hair, oops – schoolgirl, shows future promise. Rigidly ignore in case someone is watching.

Plump, flustered, badly dressed, two screaming kids. Pass - look straight ahead. She might ask for help.

Thirty or so, nice figure, long hair, smiling, oh – large man in tow. Forget it.

This is better. Nice shape, nice legs, heels. Make up. Carefully curled hair. Knees pressed tight together. Expression as if she is sucking on a lemon. Probably never had an orgasm in her life. Don't bother. Don't meet her eyes – she probably bites.

Oh, now wait a minute. What about this! Wow, watch those breasts move! Does she know what that does to me? Comfortable shape – I'll check out her butt as she passes. Love the hair. And she's got a smile in her eyes. Oh hell! I wish I could talk to her. Will she mind if I smile?

Clever, aren't they? And they do this to every woman they see, day in, day out. It is entirely automatic and you'll never stop them doing it. And it gets worse. If you take their fancy and they have time to indulge themselves, they will start wondering what you look like without your clothes. So the next time you are dressed in your best and walk into a restaurant or a cocktail party, remember that you are being X-rayed by at least half the men there and they see you walking up to the bar in the nude. Or perhaps just in stockings and garter belt. Don't worry – they are probably flattering you.

Before you scream in frustration or decide to spend the rest of your life dressed in a potato sack, reflect that men have always been like that. Only men who prefer budgerigars or other men will fail to do it. At least we have now trained them to keep their speculations to themselves and that makes relationships easier. Men have always enjoyed looking at women and still the world goes round. Don't get mad, get even and exploit the situation.

What do men think looks sexy?

People as different as men and women are bound to have different ideas about what looks sexy. Men are believed to take in a whole-body image of a woman when they first see her. If she is interesting, they register an image of her sexual features – legs, butt, breasts – and then add hair and face. Interestingly, men find it difficult to recall details of what she was wearing or the color of her eyes. They retain a strong opinion of her attractiveness but often cannot tell you much beyond whether she was wearing a skirt or pants. It is as if they are more interested in the effect of her presentation than the details of the presentation itself. A woman seeing the same person is much more likely to be able to recall what she was wearing, perhaps because her mind is unclouded by the question of sexual attractiveness.

It follows that subtlety is probably wasted on men; it will be only the obvious that stays in their minds. There is not much point worrying about the color balance of the chiffon scarf you have wound about your neck to highlight your new blouse. He might remember that you had something around your neck but he will certainly recall that the cold had made your nipples stick out like thumbs.

Women look in acid scorn at the girl at the party who has the men hanging around her like dogs at a barbecue. She is dressed just like a slut, her skirt is too short, her breasts are halfway out of her blouse, and those heels are ridiculous. But hey, she is not sitting at home on Saturday night waiting for the phone to ring. She must be doing something right.

Men in bed dream about sex. Their minds are filled not with pictures of fashion statements but erotic images of women. Of succulent thighs, rounded hips, soft and swinging breasts, heavy feminine bottoms. And that is what they find sexy when they are awake as well.

Don't Men care about Personality?

Nope. Not at first sight. An empty-headed bimbo will get as much attention as you do. Or probably more, because she survives by getting men to take care of her and she has had a lifetime of practice. But don't be depressed; it doesn't take much of a personality to catch a man but you will need one to keep him.

In the meantime, you must concentrate on understanding what men find sexy, so watch the bimbos and learn. It should not be too difficult. After all, you are smarter than they are, aren't you?

Men are so Childish!

Well, yes, I can see why you might say that, but you would be wrong. Let me give you two reasons. Firstly, heterosexual men make up nearly half of the population. If they all have similar reactions to women (and they do, believe me) then you cannot call the reactions childish. They are part of the fundamental male spirit.

The second reason is that some of the very same men have painted masterpieces, created sublime music, ruled empires and written literature that endures for centuries. Nearer to home you have devoted fathers, solid carers and servers of the community, and quiet gardeners. Inside all of them, sometimes open for view and sometimes discretely hidden, is the same old Adam who would just love to reach out and caress the waitress's bottom. It is simply the nature of the beast. You do not have to like the situation, just understand how it works.

Oh, and if you are ever feeling superior about it, run down to the newsagents or supermarket check-out and buy a women's magazine or a Mills & Boon novel. Who looks shallow and childish now?

Are you a Sex Object?

Of course you are. You are a woman, so it follows that you are a sex object. In male eyes there are no alternative positions. The only question is how successful you are at it (in his eyes). Again, you do not have to like the situation but you will have to live it.

I hope you do not feel terrible and trapped in a world you cannot change. The best response is to quietly take control of your bit of it and even out the playing field. Perhaps it will help to think of the pig-board.

Have you ever used a pig-board? Do you even know what one is? Well, the story goes like this. If you ever meet a pig face to face, you will see a dense mass of muscle on four legs. Probably not much over knee-high but as heavy as you are. This pork bulldozer is controlled by a surprisingly intelligent brain behind those piggy eyes. You will realize in an instant that if this pig wants to walk right through you, there will be nothing you can do to prevent it. So how are you going to control him? Negotiate? Tell him that his piggy way of looking at you is out-dated and that his worldview must change? Not a chance. Instead you use a pig-board.

A pig-board is a rectangle of light ply or aluminium with a handhold cut into the centre of the top edge. It is wide enough to reach across the fenced races you find in stockyards and pig farms, and high enough that the pig cannot see over it. So if you want to close off a race and divert the pig into a neighbouring pen, you merely hold the pig-board in front of your trembling knees and close off the pig's view of the open race behind you. He will then trot sweetly into the pen you have opened for him, instead of bowling you over and leaving hoof-prints over you and your little piece of ply. Magic!

Every species of animal has blind spots and the pig-board exploits the pig's natural instincts. You have a pretty good idea of what your man's natural instincts are concerning women; you just have to use your knowledge to get an even break.

- 3 -

There are no ugly women. Only lazy ones.
Helena Rubenstein

'Tisn't beauty, so to speak, nor good talk necessarily.
It's just It. Some women will stay in a man's memory if
they once walked down a street.
Rudyard Kipling

Sinking your Hook

You want to make love to your man, to give him the best he has ever had. You do not want him to imagine — ever — that he could get better loving in another woman's bed. And you want him to know that it is coming from you, that you are not acting a part or pretending but showing him what you really feel about him.

So let us get serious about what needs to be done. The first step is to attract his attention. Even if you get out of the same bed every morning and have breakfast together, you still need to focus his attention on you as a woman. Never let the pressures of work, family, running your house allow you to forget the deal you made with him — you stay with me and I'll be your woman. Not his cook or cleaner, not only the mother of his children. You have to be his sexual partner as well, and that means dusting off the skills you developed when you were trolling for men as a sappy twenty year old. And adding a few more, because you are older and wiser now. You know that even if you still had your lithe, youthful body it would not keep him satisfied for long. Any more than a beautiful face would keep his attention once he has realized there are no brains behind it.

The first step in lovemaking belongs to the woman. It is when the woman attracts the man and makes him look at her with a twinkle in his eye. So let us start by helping you do that. We will start by focusing a cold and honest eye on the way you look, and thinking about how you can look more tasty and irresistible to him.

Equipment Check

The woman who is content with her appearance has yet to be born. Even nuns have fashions and they are not purely to do with religion and practicality. At the other extreme, all super models complain that some part of their body displeases them. Have you seen any photos of Claudia Schiffer's butt? I am sure it is as elegant as the rest of her but apparently she doesn't want to include it in her portfolio.

Or look at supremely attractive women who are not strictly beautiful. Take Julia Roberts as a prime example. Men love watching her and she even starred in a blockbuster as Pretty Woman. Try to look at her in detail and you start to wonder if you would be beautiful given the same bits and pieces. Probably not. You would just look strange and gawky because her beauty comes from the inside and you do not have the character and confidence that she does. Yet.

So take it from me, nature has supplied you with what it takes to catch a man's attention. No matter if you think your nose is too long or your butt too big. No matter if you are unfortunate enough to be missing a limb or confined to a wheelchair. You have got what you need. (And even if you have managed to convince yourself that something about your body is impossibly horrid, you're stuck with it so you will have to work around it.)

This is not to say that you should not be taking good care of the equipment you have been issued with. Take care of yourself; exercise and eat sensibly, but do not imagine that because a girl feels fat and unattractive, she will automatically feel more attractive just by losing weight. You know people who are carrying a few more pounds or kilograms than they need but are still very attractive.

So take a good look at yourself in the mirror and try to honestly assess your good points and problem areas. Go ahead and make a list, but make sure that for every negative there is at least one positive. Don't just read this and think about it. I mean get pen and paper, sit down, and really make a list. It's a very important first step to recognizing yourself. This is a difficult exercise and I do not think I would trust one person in a hundred to do it successfully on their own. So get help.

A note on asking for other people's opinions. You need to find a totally trustworthy or totally disinterested male if you want an honest opinion. Your girl friends will always lie to you. And even when they are trying hard to tell the truth, they probably have less idea of what men find attractive than you do and will try to shape you in the image of women they respect – like their mother or junior school teacher. Asking your mother for advice is a non-starter unless she is a truly remarkable and hard woman. Male homosexuals are often thought to have a good appreciation of female beauty and an innate dress sense – if you know one it could be worth a try. The man you chose to trust needs to be a little artistic, honest and not too close to you. Perhaps a friend's husband (with her permission of course). And if you can get more than one opinion, so much the better.

Dressing to Capture

Why bother? Especially if you have already caught your man. Listen to me, girl. Regardless of who you dress for when you are at work or going to church, when you are with your man he wants you beside him dressed as a sexy woman. That doesn't mean that you cannot wear a tee shirt and faded jeans. It just means you have to wear the right tee shirt and the right jeans. Look at them first; if either of them fails to show off the nice shapes within, show no mercy. Into the bin they go.

Think of the checklist you made of your good and bad points, and dress accordingly. If, for instance, you have decided that your breasts are large and prominent, you need to stock up on vee-necked tops that encourage men to look down your cleavage. Or tops that are shaped around your boobs and hug you tight below them, so that your breasts are definitely your leading points. If your legs are your finest feature, then you should forget about pants for most occasions and go for skirts that are a couple of inches shorter than you're comfortable with (or six inches shorter than your mother would approve).

As a general rule, prefer skirts and dresses before pants for two reasons. Firstly, skirts are a feminine preserve and it never hurts to emphasize your femininity. Secondly, men looking at you will get the strangest feeling creeping over them. They sense that just there, just behind the curtain of your skirt, where they could reach out and touch it (if you would only let them) is the nicest thing they can think of. Better even than beer and football combined. If only you would sit a little differently, they could see it for themselves. Strange, isn't it? Men can spend a decade without ever getting to see what women hide under their skirts (unless they want them to of course), and still that little imp of an idea pops into their minds when you sit and cross your legs. And pants just don't do the same thing.

Pay attention to your underwear. A wise woman – Dorothy Parker – once said brevity is the soul of lingerie. This is definitely true if your man is going to see you wearing nothing else. But apart from those special occasions, lingerie should have the same sort of invisibility that subtle make-up has. There are exceptions of course. Perhaps you are flaunting yourself in flimsy creations that are pretty enough to be displayed through your outer clothes, but for the rest, do you really want to show everyone the visible panty line that your cheap panties carve across your buns? Or rolls of fat above and below your bra sides as they disappear behind you? Do you want people to see your comfortable, boring bra at all? If you are going to display your lingerie, make sure you are wearing something worth looking at. If not, wear something invisible.

Lingerie is an important foundation for your clothes. First, your bra. Bras are perhaps the most difficult of all clothes to design. Women and their breasts are so varied that clothing stores have to keep rack after rack after rack of bras to accommodate all the different breast sizes and textures. A typical bra is a masterpiece of dynamic engineering, probably engineered by a man but sold exclusively to women. A man will often buy sexy panties for his lady, or a see-through slip, but he is not going to risk buying a bra. No matter how it looks, she is not going to wear it unless it is comfortable, and that means trying it on first. So the racks contain what women want to wear, not what men want to see.

Women are looking for a garment to support, restrain and conceal, and the bra engineers do their best to oblige. Men think differently, because they are born with an instinctive love of breasts. They want to see as much as possible, and they want breasts to be free to move and entice them. Of course they do not have the problem of running for a bus or hurrying downstairs with wildly swinging breasts, but some form of compromise should be possible.

Bras and breasts are probably the area where male desires and female practicalities diverge most dramatically. Let's face it, what he would really, really like to see is you looking a wet tee-shirt contestant. Of course, that is not going to happen, at least, not in public. However, the fact that he is not going to get his fantasy fulfilled does not give you permission to wrap and bandage yourself up like a nun with five broken ribs. Compromise is needed if you are going to look tantalizing.

The aim is for your breasts to appear, through your blouse or sweater, as smooth, round and desirable. Forget the heavy-duty marine canvas that many bras seem to be based on. You really do not need a fabric much heavier than a nylon stocking to support yourself. There are bras on the market with cups of soft, sheer, stretchy fabric that have no seams and are tastefully see-through. Try those. Avoid cups with heavy seams or frills and gatherings that show through your clothes as a confused jumble of bumps.

As far as I know, all women have nipples but all of us are a little coy about the impression they make through our clothes when we are cold (or excited!). A silly little worry, I know, but there it is. Or was, because times are changing and other women no longer object to seeing enticing little buttons (of course, men have never had any difficulty with the idea). A recent episode of *Sex in the City* even featured nipple enhancements, small, pointed disks that sit over your nipples and make them appear more prominent. Interesting, but I hope you do not find one of them slipping out of place. That would be very confusing.

And then there are the ladies who are convinced that their breasts are too small. If you have ever visited Asia and gone into an up-market department store, you will have been astounded at the rows and rows of rigid points on the bra racks. They look like little white anti-aircraft missiles. Each pair is well padded and when they are worn the effect is like two ice-cream cones. The ladies who sport these monstrosities usually have the sort of lithe, youthful figures that we in the West would sell our souls for. Too small? They must be joking! Most Westerners have not had breasts like that since they were sixteen, and would just love to have them again.

If you have been issued with small breasts, your best tactic is not to pad and bandage but to show them off with minimum or no restraint. Concentrate on showing off shape and movement. Don't be too shy to wear no bra under your tee shirt. Your only problem in public will be trying not to laugh when the men trip over their tongues.

As with bras, so with panties and panty hose. It's hopeless to wear an elegantly crafted pair of pants if underneath you have panties or tights that bundle your buns up into a shapeless bolster behind you. There are tights designed to fit women whose butts are in two halves (a feature that is not as rare as some panty hose designers seem to think) and these are the ones to look for. Wolfords of Europe (www.wolford.com) make some especially fetching designs. Their Fatal range looks as if you have had glitter sprayed on you whilst nude, and they are sheer all the way to the top. That will raise his temperature!

Your butt is a major erotic attraction to men, and you should take care of it. The thong panty has come to the rescue recently and made the sight of retreating women a real sensual experience for men. Now, I know there are women who find them uncomfortable. I can understand that but believe me, they are something you can get used to if you want to. And besides, as the old French saying goes 'To be beautiful, you must suffer'. If they get just too irritating, they don't take up much room in your purse. The feeling of freedom and naughtiness they give is very stimulating.

The effect you are looking for is one that draws the male eye to your sexy features. To do this you have to be obvious, probably much more obvious than you feel comfortable with. Never mind; you will know you have got the level of provocation about right when a female friend suggests you are looking too sexy. Tell her that no one ever lost a man's attention by looking too sexy.

Cosmetic Assistance

Should you wear make-up? Now that's not a simple question. Mostly it depends on what you are doing. If you are mucking out your stables, a full paint job is clearly uncalled for, but you might feel happier with just a touch of lipstick and shadow. I don't suppose the horses will care but you never know who might come by...

Most women who use make-up regularly feel naked without it. On the other hand, where I live – in the humid tropics – making up is a battle that many women have already lost. They don't wear a lick of make-up from one year to the next. That is a shame because they are missing out on a great aid. No matter who you are or what you look like, artful make-up can say a lot about you. The trick is to have different cosmetic schemes for different occasions. Too many ladies use just one scheme, and whether they are going to work, a wedding or a funeral, the same one has to cover all situations.

No matter how you present yourself at work, for other occasions you definitely need a make-up scheme that is overtly sexy. Go to a beautician that you trust and tell them you need something that will make men sit up and beg. Take magazine pictures that express the statement you want to make. They might not suit you in detail (everyone has their own colors), but they will give the beautician an idea of the heat you wish to generate. You probably need two stages; one scheme that just looks sexy, and another that pulls out all the stops and warns the world that tonight your demons have taken over.

Crowning Glory

Listen very carefully: men like long hair. Men like long hair. Men like long hair. Men like long hair. Men like long hair. Men like long hair. Men like long hair. Men like long hair. Men like long hair. Men like long hair. Men like long hair. Men like long hair. Men like long hair. Men like long hair. Men like long hair. Men like long hair. Men like long hair. Men like long hair. Men love long hair.

It's true. If you ran an opinion poll with more than two males sampled, you would get a majority vote for long hair. Long hair is fundamentally feminine and a clear signal to the interested male. Long hair is beautiful in itself and adds to your beauty. Long hair feels erotic to him, especially on his naked skin. Your long hair draped over the pillow is one of the world's most erotic images.

Even that famous old priest from Germany, Martin Luther – hardly noted for his devotion to the erotic life – said 'Hair is the richest ornament of women'.

If you would ever like to display your charms in a girlie magazine, you will find that the one requirement the photo editor has before he will check the pneumatic beauty of your intimate assets is – long hair. He knows that men buy girlie magazines, and – men like long hair.

Sure long hair is inconvenient sometimes and needs more care, but on the plus side you can do more things with long hair. You can wear it up or wear it down, plaits, ponytail, French roll – you name it. You can't do all those things with hair like a man's, can you?

So why do we see so many women with short hair? Of course, there are women who just do not care what men think of them, so they are free to cut their hair as they like. Then there are the ladies who feel that curled and permed hair makes them look more distinguished or business-like, and that is more important to them than pleasing any man. (I don't know if hair like that will make you look more business-like, but I can guarantee it will put an instant 10 years on your appearance.)

The other causal factor is that when women get their hair done, they ask their friends how it looks. I'm sure your friends have asked your opinion. And what did you say? "Oh, it's wonderful. It makes you look just like your mother." Or perhaps "It's so brave of you to cut your hair short like that. You look just like a coconut on a stick." Of course you did not. You said "That's really nice – pretty – wonderful – so refreshing – I wish I could do the same" etc etc. I can understand you. Little white lies make the world go round, and besides, if one of your friends disfigures herself in the name of fashion, that is just one less competitor, isn't it?

What is really shameful about your lack of honesty is that you probably asked your friends the same question and you believed the answer! Shame on you!

Of course, you do not have to believe me. Just bear it in mind when you take your man for the Mall Test below.

Oh, and just in case you've forgotten – MEN LIKE LONG HAIR.

The Mall Test

Perhaps by now you are feeling a little battered and you need to get your feet back on the ground, take a dose of reality, hop back out of the looking glass. Perhaps it's a good time to take The Mall Test. This is quite simple. Lead your man off to a busy mall café and order a couple of cappuccinos. Sit out in front of the café, side by side, and watch the world go by.

The object of the test is to see if you can predict your man's reactions to the women passing by. Of course you will have to let him off the leash a little and reassure him that favourable comments about other women are permitted – for the duration of the test at least. You might have to convince him that you are not trying to trap him and you are not storing up ammunition for future use. Try to avoid saying things like 'But I have a pair of culottes just like that and you said you liked them!' Just listen to what he is saying and remember what he likes.

If you think he is holding back and not telling you what he really thinks, try him on the Thong Panty Game. This involves watching the approaching women and predicting whether they are wearing thong panties or the old fashioned, cut-your-buns-in-two type. Two points for a correctly predicted thong, one for predicting old-fashioned panties, and minus one for a mistake. I hope that your man scores better than you do, although as your skills improve you might be able to beat him. Anyway, it will break the ice and you should be able to get what you really want – a picture of what excites him about women. I am sure you will end up finding that his interests are simpler and more basic than even you had expected.

Once you have a clear picture of his inner preferences, what do you do next? Why, use the knowledge against him, of course; but that starts a new chapter.

- 4 -

Trust me, Paulette, you have all the equipment.
You just need to read the manual.
Elle Woods in Legally Blonde

God gave women intuition and femininity. Used properly, the
combination easily jumbles the brain of any man I've ever met.
Farrah Fawcett

Lovemaking – the First Steps

Armed with your new and perhaps jaundiced view of the way men think, you can start thinking about how it affects your lovemaking. It is best to begin at the beginning and ask yourself when lovemaking actually starts, when do you light the fuse? And of course, how long it should last? According to that well-known epicure and savant Johnny Rotten of the Sex Pistols, love is two minutes fifty-two seconds of squishing noises. Maybe for him, but not for you. You definitely want more than that. So how much would you settle for? Five minutes? Ten minutes? Twenty minutes sounds better or even half an hour on special occasions.

You will have to lift your sights if you want to become a courtesan of legend. Even a quickie against the wall of the fitting room at Victoria's Secret starts long before. Hours before, if you can manage it. You are not thinking on a male time scale. A woman might say to her lover 'Take me to bed and make passionate love to me. Kiss me, stroke me, caress me. Give me orgasm after orgasm until I faint from ecstasy.   And then bring me garlic mushrooms and bacon for breakfast, with orange juice and real coffee'.

It doesn't work that way for your man. Practically speaking, he is limited to a single miserly orgasm and that doesn't take very long to achieve. For Johnny Rotten it apparently takes only two minutes fifty-two seconds. If he is to have a full grape-to-champagne experience, it has to start long before you have taken off your clothes and reached for each other's interesting bits.

And given that you are bringing the intelligence to the enterprise, initiating and controlling the whole performance is in your hands. You need to catch your man's attention and tease and provoke him. Give him thrills of anticipation and then close the door on him for a while. Hint at what you could give him if you felt like it. Caress his mind and body and keep him in a state of stimulation. The longer you keep him on edge before the end run, the more he will love you.

Time enough

When you decide to make a move on your man, you need to be reasonably sure that you can control the next few hours of his time. Although dancing around in a G-string half an hour before the Super Bowl is not a complete waste of time, the looming kick-off will limit your options. (Dancing around in a G-string is never a waste of time. At least he will not confuse you with anyone else. I hope.)

It doesn't hurt to demand his time. Ask him if he has anything special on for the rest of the day. Persuade him that he has nothing important and then say something like "Good – because I have something special you can do for me when we get back from shopping".

Try to pick a time – say Saturday afternoon – when all you both have planned is a trip to the shops or similar, and an evening at home. If you have kids, make sure their plans do not conflict with yours. It's difficult for a mother, but sometimes your man deserves to come first. It's vital for your relationship that he doesn't always have to accept second place. As a group, we are notorious for self-sacrifice. We routinely give up everything for our families. But are we giving up on our relationship as well?

Once they arrive, kids will stay in your house for fifteen years or more; you can't expect your man to be content with hurried, silent quickies in your darkened bedroom for fifteen years straight. Sometimes you just have to farm the kids out, drop them with your mother, have them sleep over, do whatever you can. And once they have left you alone for a few hours, forget them. It's your man's turn for all your attention and if you keep reaching for the phone to check on them, you will be curdling whatever magic you manage to stir up.

Never go swimming on a full stomach

And never make love on one either. The best thing to do with a full stomach is sleep it off, and going to bed to sleep is not what you are aiming at. A light lunch is indicated. And preferably no alcohol – yet.

Just as you don't want your man surfeited on food, you don't want him to be suffering from a surplus of recent lovemaking either. Ideally, he should not have made love for 24 – 48 hours. More than this and he might not be able to withstand your teasing for long enough: less than this and he will not admire your efforts with the same appreciation.

Dress Well, and You are On!

Remember – emphasize your best (sexiest) features. Show off bits that would upset the minister. Aim for an appearance on the tarty side of elegant. Push your limits a little – if you are feeling comfortable with what you are wearing, it probably means you are not trying hard enough. Dab of make-up, straighten up the stockings, whatever – you know what needs to be done.

Once you are ready, it's Showtime!

Picture yourself coming out of the bedroom, ready to go. He is sitting waiting for you (how did I guess?), idly flicking through the television channels until you are ready. You trot in looking very tasty and say...

What do you say to set the scene? Definitely not "I wonder how the kids are?" or "Did you remember to bring those discount vouchers for the dog food?" You are about to start making love to him, and cheap dog food doesn't enter the equation. How about "I'm sorry, Honey, but I can't get this skirt right. I think it's just too long. What do you think?"

Don't be upset if he can't respond sensibly. That just means that you have not trained him well enough in the past – although things are going to change in the future. You may just have to carry on with your next lines by yourself.

"I think it would be much better like this, don't you?" and hold the hem up to a more attractive level. "Come on – let's go and buy a more sexy one. I feel like living dangerously."

Of course, it doesn't have to be your skirt; it could be your bra, or your top or whatever. As long as you both leave the house with the intention of doing something to make you look even sexier.

You were standing at the top of the mountain, and you just uncrossed your skis and pushed yourself off. You are really going to enjoy the ride!

Have Fun

What is shopping to a man? Park the car, troll slowly around the supermarket, steer an overloaded trolley through the checkout and back to the car. Go home, watch television.

So once he has parked the car, put your hand (note the pretty varnished fingernails) on his thigh and say "Screw the shopping, Honey. I'll do it tomorrow. Let's go and have fun." It's possible he might resist. His Conscience and Protestant Work Ethic might force you to beg a little, but I don't think you will be forced to throw yourself on the ground and kick your heels in a tantrum.

How do you have fun together? I hope for your sake that it doesn't mean visiting one of those pokey little shops that sell model trains. That would be a challenge. Try and waylay him into a café or a food centre, but pick somewhere with a view of the world. Eating and drinking together is a basic human ritual. It is the way that humans reinforce their bonds, and taking a coffee together is about more than just drinking coffee. You could have stayed at home and made yourself a cup of instant if that was all there was to it. If you have not had lunch, now is a good time to take it – a light lunch, remember? Tell him to just have a snack because you want to eat later.

Time to Tease

While you are sitting and watching the world go by, start to steer his thoughts in the right direction. Talk about the eligible women walking past. Specifically, talk about their naughty bits. Criticize the way they are not making the most of their assets. Complain if someone is wearing an ugly bra, compliment a nicely displayed ass. Ask him if he thinks they would be a good lay – as if you would ever let him find out for real. Wonder out loud how that elegant businesswoman looks as she reaches a climax. Ask him intimate questions about sex with other women, how did they look when they came? Ask him how you look as you slip out of control.

Your aim is to get him thinking about sex, about boobs and butts, the nice, naughty, wobbly bits. Specifically yours, of course, but there is no harm in starting with other girls' attractions. You might even learn something from his reactions.

Then shut him down for a while and go and do something else together. What? That depends on what you like doing together, and on what is available. Go swimming – you needed to buy new swimming things anyway (if you dare to buy a one-piece, I will throw this book at you. Unless it doesn't have a back, of course). I have seen a shopping centre with a bungee jumping deck over the swimming pool – that would be fun and different. Or go to the travel agent and review an ideal holiday – it can't hurt to dream, can it?

While you are with him, keep touching him. Lean against him, pat his butt, brush your breast against his arm – all unconsciously of course. You should be breathing some life into him by now so respond to any touching you get in return. If he pats your butt, wiggle it and purr. When a pussycat purrs, it is likely to get stroked some more.

Lighting the Fire

Do not let him forget that he agreed to help you buy a new short skirt (or bra or whatever you settled on back home). It's time to lead him off to the most suitable boutique. Now a well-trained male has no difficulty helping his woman buy interesting clothes. If yours thinks that buying clothes is a purely female occupation, I guess you've been mishandling him. You need to have him beside you picking out a suitable garment, and you need to get him into the fitting room with you. This is most important because you want him to think of you as a sex symbol, and to help display your charms at their best. You want his sexual enthusiasm to help shape the way you are going to dress. You want him to feel every time you step out in your new sexy top 'That's my woman and I made her show off her boobs like that'.

Are you despairing of getting your man into the fitting room? Well, you should have trained him better. However, life was not meant to be easy and you will just have to use all the wiles you can muster. Try bribery (men are always more comfortable being bribed than blackmailed). "Buy me something else as well, Honey. I promise I'll wear it for you, no matter what it is." If that doesn't get him interested, you really have a problem.

When you get to the fitting room, sit him down and get him comfortable while you do a striptease for him. Don't bundle clothes up under your arms to try others on; take them off and show off the lingerie you have put on for him. Get him to help, even if hooking and unhooking bras are mysteries beyond male understanding. Above all, get his opinion on what you are buying. You will have to be diplomatic especially if this is his first time fitting you up with sexy clothes. Don't cry and say 'But that's just for teenagers! I'm too old….' Suffer in silence; after all, he might well be right.

All the time you are playing in the fitting room, remember you are trying to tease and provoke him – but not to satisfy him. Not at this time, anyway. Do outrageous things. Gauge his level of interest in the clothes by patting his erection. Do a little lap dance for him once you get down to bra and panties. Pull the skirt around your butt, say you can see a panty line and shuck your panties off. Hang them behind the door and leave them there. Keep asking him if the new clothes are sexy enough to get him hard. If necessary, send him out to get more clothes.

When you leave, joke with the attendant about how hot and horny you are going to look in your new clothes, and what will probably happen to you as a result. As you leave the store tell him how naughty you feel having left your panties behind the fitting room door. Describe how nice it feels having your skirt swish across your bottom.

Even the dumbest male will have realized by now that something good is going on, and that the rest of the day promises to be very interesting. And there we will leave him for the moment.

- 5 -

According to a new survey, women say they feel more comfortable undressing in front of men than they do undressing in front of other women. They say that women are too judgmental where, of course, men are just grateful.
Robert De Niro

There is no excellent beauty that hath not some strangeness in the proportion.
Francis Bacon

What's on Offer?

Until now we have been concentrating on how you use dress sense to enhance your sex appeal, but at some point the clothes will be coming off – most of them anyway – and you'll be left with nothing to hide behind. Are you worried? Well, you shouldn't be.

So – let's get down to it and I need your active participation here. (Sitting and reading about it will not work; we are dealing with deep-seated prejudices here, so be a good girl for once and do what I ask). Stand in front of your biggest mirror naked, and what do you see? A Playboy centerfold? A glamorous porn star? A wild and exotic woman with a body men would die for? If you see any of them, perhaps you don't need this book. My husband says just autograph it with your phone number and send it in for a refund; he'll get back to you.

In the real world, standing in the mirror will be just you, warts and all. You have seen yourself like this a million times and if you ever stopped to look more closely, your reaction was probably 'Oh God, I wish I wasn't so fat!' It's just your body and you have been living in it for a touch more than sixteen years; all your life in fact. Of course it looks ordinary to you.

Fortunately, your man doesn't have the same attitude. For a man, the chance to see your body is a privilege, something to be treasured. No matter how many times he has seen it before, he likes looking at you. When he is hungry and you are sending out sexy thoughts, he will look at you with more naked desire than a starving man watching a dripping steak come off the barbecue.

Through his Eyes

Back to the mirror and let's try and imagine how he sees you. You want to look your best, so try softening the lights. No one looks good in a fluorescent glare. Now comb your hair. Try swishing it from side to side; it looks good in the soft light, doesn't it?

Are you wearing any jewellery? Take time out to put some on, and while you are at it, freshen your make up. Don't forget the nail varnish, toes as well. How are you looking now? Admit it, you're looking more interesting and you feel a bit more comfortable standing nude in front of the mirror. To him, you will be looking more tasty, not because you have painted your toes but because you are feeling happier about yourself. Look at yourself more closely; strike poses for the fun of it. Hold your hands over your head and pirouette. Looking good? As far as he's concerned, you already look tastier than that steak.

Moving on and down we start to get to the more sensitive bits. Specifically, your breasts. Breasts are powerful symbols of femininity. Deep in the human psyche the female breast means all the good and bountiful things about women and motherhood. In primitive art, the Earth Mother was portrayed with a variable number of breasts, multiplying her magical powers. What would men have done if their women really had so many breasts? Perhaps we can guess. Men have not progressed very far; they are still in awe of the female breast, and the more they can play with them, the happier they feel. They don't want to think about them; just lick them.

While men have very clear ideas about breasts and what to do with them, modern Western women have a confused picture of their breasts. On the one hand they treasure their femininity and the ability to feed babies and give life. On the other hand, they recognize what potent sexual symbols they carry on their chests, and they are just a little scared of them.

Imagine passing through a city train or bus station. Sitting on one of the benches, a young mother is feeding her baby. Natural, beautiful to some, slightly embarrassing to others, but the world doesn't come to a halt. Even in the West such an image presents no challenge. Now erase the baby from the picture and leave the young lady sitting unconcernedly on the bench with her breasts exposed. What a nightmare scenario we have created now! You can imagine situations when you might just breast feed in public; you may even have done it on occasion. It would take world revolution, a million dollars and a large bottle of wine to make you just sit in the bus station and show off your precious breasts to the passers-by.

Right now, standing in front of the mirror, your feelings about your breasts are not important. What you want to know is how he feels about them, and you will be pleased to know that men's attitude to breasts is extremely simple. Breasts exist for men to play with, nothing more. Men love them; they love their roundness and their softness. They love their shape and their femaleness. They love to watch them, and to see them move and change shape as you work in the kitchen. They love to touch them and cup them with their hands. Tease the nipples into peaks and listen to your sighs as they do it.

If you push them into it, they might admit to preferring this pair to that pair but ask them if they would like you to leave your top off on the beach or perhaps wear a soft blouse with no bra to dinner, there will not be a millisecond of hesitation. Men love breasts so much that any pair will satisfy them, even yours.

Look at them in the mirror and try hard to imagine you are a sixteen year-old schoolboy looking at his first pair of breasts. Imagine how much in awe he would be of you, and how he would be dying to reach out and touch them. Now you are beginning to think like a man! Tease your nipples until they stand up. That looks provocative. Try standing in part profile so you see the shape of your breast with the nipple at its peak; he would love that. Lift your arms up and watch the shape change. Cup your breasts and offer them to the mirror. How could he resist you?

Moving Down

Now comes the bit that is responsible for more female depression than any other part of your anatomy. You might have a firm, flat, athletic middle; I am told such ladies exist although I don't look like that and neither do any of my friends. Probably you are more like the other 98% of the female population who are best described as soft and yielding.

Stand sideways on to your mirror. If you can look across your tummy from hipbone to hipbone, then your tummy is perfectly flat. The question is, do you want it to be perfectly flat? No man is going to want to climb into bed with an anorexic skeleton, and most of them would be a little cautious about a highly muscled distance runner or ballet dancer. They want women who have soft round tummies. When a man takes a woman to bed, softness and generosity are part of the attraction.

Of course, you can have too much of a good thing. A tummy that sticks out more than your breasts or – worse still – forces you to sit with your legs open, is definitely too much of a good thing. Very well, you will have to put up with it for the moment, but you are going to have to do something about it in the longer term. I can't suggest anything other than boring old diet and exercise, but I can give you a tip. When you start out on your figure modification program, put your bathroom scales in the closet and get yourself a tape measure instead. You don't care how much you weigh; what you are interested in is how you look. Check your progress by measuring the important bits. Working out in the gym can tone up the muscles of your stomach and thighs, and slim your waist, without making much difference to your weight. After a couple of months you can be looking svelte, sexy and cat-like but still weigh pretty much the same. By the same token, if you try to change your shape by diet alone and skip the exercise, you can go from being too big, heavy and flabby to being slightly smaller, lighter and still just as flabby. Not what you want to show your man.

But that's all in the future; right now you are who you are and you will have to play the cards in your hand. Just avoid standing sideways on to him.

Lovely Legs

Women's legs are not the same as men's legs. I am sure you have noticed. Where men's legs tend to be strong and heavily muscled (and hairy), women's are naturally slimmer and they look longer. For once, this is not just a myth; in proportion to their body, women's legs actually are slightly longer.

As you look in the mirror, stand with your feet about a foot (30 cm) apart. Standing this way, your legs will appear more or less straight all the way down. (In fact your thighbones start at your hips and are inclined towards each other. If you are skinny enough you might be able to see this.) Unlike men, it is rare (and not particularly attractive) to be able to clearly see the muscles of a woman's thighs, although her calf muscles give interesting curves. Your biggest enemy – again – is fat. It's easy to put fat on to your thighs and if there is too much, your thighs rub together and you can look ponderous. Oh dear – diet and exercise again! So get out the mountain bike or the cross-country skis and go and conquer a few hills.

Unlike the tummy problem, you do have quick fixes for legs. Do you have high heels? Run and get them, and stand in front of the mirror again just as you were. You look better already; your legs have got longer. The next step is to slip on panty hose or stockings. Now you are looking even sexier as they smooth out the dubious areas. Not that making love in panty hose is recommended (it makes your toes curl) but standing in front of the mirror wearing tights and heels does show you that even difficult thighs can be presented in a flattering light. Is this cheating? Not at all. Sex is like magic; the trick is not to saw the lady in half but to make your audience think she has been sawn in half. But now take the panty hose off again; there is more to be checked out.

And round the Back?

There are men's magazines and many websites devoted solely to admiration of the female butt. Strange? Not really. Just as male eyes always drop to your breasts when they see the front of you, so they drop to admire your butt when you cannot see what they are looking at. You like to see firm male buns – for many women they are the only things that make football tolerable – so you can understand that he likes to look at women from that point of view.

How are you blessed in that department? It is difficult to make a real judgment by looking over your shoulder; all that twisting round distorts your butt and your view. You will need another mirror to see behind you. Again, remember that you are trying to look with his eyes. For him a fine, female bottom has to be obvious. Large and shapely. It can be muscular and stick out behind, like an ice-skater's, or it can be heavy and pear-shaped like that of a mature courtesan. A firm, slim, androgynous bottom that might belong to a young girl or boy can make it to the fashion catwalk but that's not what men crave. They want something to pat and to hold. Something comfortable to sit on their lap, and if it doesn't wobble a little as you walk, they'll be disappointed.

Whatever shape you have been given, as long as it is prominent and female he will be interested. This is an area where a certain amount of fat is essential. Not a gross excess, of course, but you've already decided to get out your mountain bike for the thighs and stomach, haven't you?

A nice round female bottom is just made to be patted and by Heavenly design, each half fits comfortably in a man's hand. Mmh; you shouldn't argue with that.

The Sacred Bit

At the base of your stomach – your nicely rounded stomach – is your mons or pubic mound. Tucked under your mons and between the tops of your thighs is the thing that defines a woman. You can get by with not much in the way of breasts or long straight legs. A man can accept a small muscular butt or even (shudder) short hair. But your pussy is the ultimate demonstration of your femininity. Without it, who are you?

This is the biggest secret, the Holy of Holies, the Well at the End of the World. It is the Mount Pleasant at the end of the male pilgrim's journey. It is the inspiration for much of the world's art and most of its stories. Hollywood could have no romance or heroines if there were no pussies to drive the story line. Even Mickey Mouse had to have Minnie beside him, and she had to be female, not merely a buddy.

No matter that you keep it hidden away and hardly any male ever gets to touch or even see it, your pussy's presence colours every interaction between you and men. It is the ultimate source of your sexual attraction. No boyfriend would ever hold your hand if you didn't have a pussy to entice him with. If women had penises to pee with and laid eggs like chickens, men would be lost. How would they live without their icon? Would they bother to talk to you at all?

Standing in front of the mirror, there is not much to see. Nature has conspired to hide your pussy away. Two lips either side of a furrow disappearing underneath you. Even now, with your clothes off, it is hiding away. In fact it is so well hidden that many women have not really examined themselves and are uncertain of what their man sees when he finally manages to prize their knees apart. I am sure you are not so Victorian, but we will deal with that in another chapter.

If you have had the chance to see lots of naked girl friends, or even just pictures of girls in magazines, you will have seen that pussies are almost as variable as faces. Try visiting the beaches of Greece and you'll be surprised. Each one is unique. Your man could almost certainly identify you from a photograph, so be careful next time you star in a pornographic picture movie with your girl friends; wearing a mask will not be enough.

Does your man like your pussy? Here I can say unreservedly YES! Even though there are so many different pussies in the world, fat ones, thin ones, all sorts of colours, inner petals that burst out or are discretely hidden, tiny clits or ones as fat as your pinky, men do not seem to have definite opinions on what a pretty pussy looks like. I suspect they are so much in awe of your magic purse that they do not dare to have opinions. So your man loves your pussy, and would be happy to feast on it whenever you allow him the privilege.

Forget what you think about your pussy; your opinion just doesn't matter. The great thing is to look at yourself as your man would look at you, so what does he see? Lots of hair? Oh dear!

In the 21st century most sexually aware women do something to control body hair. When did you last see a lady with tufts of hair under her arms walking the summer streets of America? Underarm hair is totally unacceptable so off it comes, without fail. The same for hairy legs; who wants to sport a mat of hair under their elegant nylons?

Attitudes to bikini hair have taken a while to catch up. Fashionable ladies were prepared to leave it to grow naturally, or at most give it a quick trim with their nail scissors. They justified their laziness on the grounds that 'no one sees it'. The fact that their man was included under 'no one' escaped their notice. To put him further in his place, they used to trim or remove any hair that might show when they wore their bikini to the beach. They wanted to look civilized for everyone else, but the one person who really cared for their pussy did not matter.

Not good enough. Your man thinks your pussy is at least as important as his face, and you wouldn't let him get away with letting his beard grow just however it wants, would you? Certainly not; he has to shave every morning. True there must be some well-loved men with wild beards, but for most of them it is an outward sign that no one cares what they look like anymore. I hope you don't think the same way about your pussy!

Unless you and your man have a particular look in mind, there are just two styles you can opt for; either naked lips with a small trimmed patch on your mons, or just naked, no hair at all. Take your pick. Your man will love you for it and you will be surprised by the results. You will look and feel cleaner, and he will like that. He will be able to see more of you, and the more he sees, the hotter he gets. He will feel you are much smoother and that makes licking you more fun. And finally you will be able to rub your pussy over his most sensitive bits for much longer before he explodes – more about that later.

So how to get yourself in shape? Well, you can shave. This is the most basic system of hair removal and it has disadvantages. First, it is much more complicated than shaving under your arms. Your pussy is much more intricate and although shaving your mound is easy, the soft and tricky bits underneath are very difficult. Especially because they are 'round the corner' and out of sight. It is next to impossible to get the bits right at the back.

The biggest drawback to shaving is the regrowth. A few hours later and you are already getting a little prickly. You might also be troubled by itching and ingrown hairs. I am afraid that shaving is for masochists only.

There are a variety of machines that roll over your skin and pull the hairs out by their roots. These are quite successful in the places you can reach easily, and as each hair is completely removed rather than cut, it regrows with a soft point. But still, the further you go out of sight, the more difficult it gets to catch all the hairs. And it might bring tears to your eyes.

Of the temporary treatments, the Rolls Royce is a Brazilian Wax at a cosmetic salon. At first thought, the idea of waxing your tender pussy and yanking the hairs out by the roots sounds like a medieval torture but the pain is instantaneous and bearable. Certainly a skilled operator will leave you completely clean front to back and you will love the smooth, silky feeling. And everyone loves the idea of lying back and having her pussy pampered. The only thing to remember is that you should not trim your hair for at least three weeks before you go for your waxing.

A practical, cheaper alternative is hair-removing cream. This you can buy in the supermarket and it is easy to use. Follow the instructions on the box (including doing a trial patch the day before) and in around 15 minutes you can have a smooth, luxurious pussy with as much or as little hair in your small patch as you want. Don't forget to go all the way back to get every hair you can find and, most importantly, make sure that any hair you leave on your mons is well clear of your lips. (We will talk about why you should do this in another chapter.)

A practical tip. If you want to craft your little patch of hair into something interesting – like a heart – you will find a secret weapon in your kitchen. It's your set of cookie cutters. Take the one you fancy and press it against your mons while you apply the hair removing cream. This is much, much better than trying to do it freehand.

All of the methods above are temporary but the best news of the new century is that you can now buy inhibiting creams. In their constant search for a solution to male baldness, the scientists accidentally came across ways of slowing hair growth. Now you can buy creams or oils to rub on your freshly cleaned skin, and the regrowth will be very slow. Results vary from person to person but for some people the cream not only slows regrowth right down, but the regrowth is soft and sparse, like baby hair. For some lucky girls there is hardly any regrowth again – ever. Magic! Try a new cream called 'Marzena' – this is very quick acting and has removing cream and inhibitor combined.

There are continual developments in the battle against unwanted hair, and I have not even mentioned permanent methods like electrolysis (well established) or laser treatment (less well known.). Try looking at www.hairfacts.com, www.folica.com or www.hairnomore.com to learn more.

The important thing about removing your hair is that your man is the only other person who is going to see it. You are giving him a present, a beautiful, well-tended pussy to play with. It shows you are thinking about your pussy as something very special, and he will enjoy the fact that you are treating it as seriously as he does.

Being Primitive

Now try this. Stand with your legs together and your back to the mirror. Keeping your legs straight, bend over as far as you can – hands flat on the floor if you can reach that far. Now look at the picture in the mirror. Your pussy is peeping and smiling through the diamond shaped window at the top of your thighs. It's as if you have been designed specifically to show it off this way.

Many millions of years ago, when humanoid ape-men were just deciding to walk on two legs, this is the favourite view they would have had of their women. When a woman wanted sex she would have lifted her tail end up into the air and waved it at the man she wanted to mount her.

It may surprise you to know that men have not lost their instinctive reaction to the sight. If you don't believe me, try doing it to the next group of building workers who whistle at you on the street – but don't complain to me if you get more than you expected! It is still a very, very provocative sight. A naked woman with her tail in the air is an instantaneous turn-on and an invitation to any man. It really is a primitive process because, viewed like that, you are nothing more than a pussy on legs. Your breasts are out of the equation, not to mention your brains, personality and all the other things that make you a warm, loveable person. You don't need to be pretty or have a delicate waist. You don't even need a shapely butt, because stretched like this they all look good. You just need a warm and tasty pussy and, thank God, every lady is issued with one of those at birth.

Now you know about this piece of magic, use it carefully

And What Else?

So, what did the mirror on the wall tell you? That you are the fairest of them all? Almost certainly not, and if you were fool enough to believe it, you would be insufferable. Mirrors do not tell you anything; they merely reflect the prejudices of the people looking into them. You might see plain old you, but he will see whatever you present him. If you are feeling fairly comfortable with the sexy body the Good Lord gave you, then that is what he will see. A bed of wild flowers fit for a man to roll in.

- 6 -

Discontented women dream of being rescued by Prince Charming.
Discontented men dream of finding a horny blond
in the back seat of a taxi.
Mason Cooley

If you've got them by the balls, their heart
and mind will follow.
John Wayne

Turning up the Heat

As I recall, we left you and your man at the boutique door after buying clothes designed to make you look even sexier, and to raise his temperature to boiling point. Your aim is to keep the sexual pot simmering for a while before you let him take your clothes off. What are you going to do with him now?

It's a funny thing about our society but there are hardly any public facilities for couples to enjoy their favorite hobby – making love. If you enjoy skating, there are ice-rinks. Glitzy sports shops sell everything from running shoes to riding helmets. You can shoot in pistol clubs; play golf on a variety of courses. Adult education centers run painting schools, massive complexes are devoted to ten-pin bowling, public libraries let us read books free of charge. And for lovers? Where are the discreet gardens where you can enjoy a bottle of wine and your lover's kisses in a shaded bower? Where are the dance clubs that insist on you checking in your outer clothes so you can show off your new lingerie? How about a restaurant for couples with soft music and young, fit waiters and waitresses wearing nothing more than miniscule, transparent g-strings as they serve you in darkened, candle-lit booths? The gym gets your body into shape, but who shows you what to do with it? Why do cinemas have films of the most gruesome violence and horror, but even the most romantic of films are not allowed to show more than a quick flash of nipple. You are much more likely to see a loaded gun in a romantic film than an erect penis.

It seems as if people – or at least the city fathers – conspire to pretend that lovemaking doesn't exist outside the bedroom. Sure they might allow a furtive sex-shop in a run-down area – but it will be a sex shop, not a love shop. There is nowhere that you can take your man that is intended to make you both feel sexy and romantic. So you're on your own and your fertile imagination will have to fill the gap.

What you are trying to do is gently stroke the warm, erotic feeling in your man's mind. He will enjoy it, of course, and it will also stoke the fire for when you finally get home.

Going to Sexy Places

Is there any naughty place in your town that you would really like to see inside? Can you persuade him to take you to a titty bar or buy you a lap dance? What? Me? Go into a place like that? Well, your main reason for going is curiosity. Don't tell me you've never wondered what actually happens in places like that (unless you've visited them before, of course). Anyone who enjoys sex wants to know what the rest of the world does, even if they don't want to join in.

The other reason for visiting a girly bar is because it will be a big turn-on for your man to escort you in. For lots of reasons. Doing something that is definitely naughty with you in public will feel very exciting. He will also enjoy your associating with girls who have a terrible reputation. (99.9% undeserved of course; they might not be bank managers or have Degrees in Advanced Librarianship, but would you want to go partying with people like that anyway?) You will earn his respect by standing tall and just taking it in your stride. If you can manage some active enjoyment as well, that's even better. Everyone appreciates a 'woman of the world'. Think of what he will feel when you say 'Take me inside. I want to see everything, but don't leave me alone!'

The whole idea might sound very uncomfortable, but in reality you will find it is all very tame and gentle, and not at all embarrassing. What the bars are like will depend on your city fathers (bless their miserable puritan hearts!). Some of them are so miserable and so puritan that they will allow no girly bars at all and you'll either have to drive to the next jurisdiction or save it for another day. In other places (mostly overseas) literally anything goes from live sex to girls shooting ping pong balls across the stage by popping them into their pussies and squeezing hard (don't you wish you had muscles like that?) In the mining town where I live, girls dance in the local pub six nights a week. The town council insists that they wear enough to cover their pussies, and pasties – small sticky patches to cover their nipples. (Who are the people who make these dumb rules? Do they imagine that the pub goers are going to be turned into slavering beasts by the sight of a nipple, while looking at the rest of the girl's breast is mild and acceptable? Don't get me started! I don't think they should be forced to retain their g-strings either. Perhaps I should go into politics.)

However much the girls are allowed to show, the whole idea of the bar is to make you feel good, take your money and attract you back again so they can take some more. The biggest danger is not that you will feel horribly uncomfortable, but that you will find it pleasantly naughty to be playing at the top of the slippery slope your mother told you about. As you walk in, it will probably be a bit dark, and there will be more men than women at the bar. That's no surprise; most bars are like that anyway. Usually there is a stage for the girls to dance on, unless this is just a topless bar where the girls serve beer and offer you the chance to admire their breasts. If there is dancing, the quality will probably be – what shall we say – ordinary? Uninspiring? Sorry, but it is difficult to be red hot night after night. Some clubs have an amateur night that can be fun; the dancers might not be so professional but they certainly enjoy themselves. The only question you might have is why men enjoy watching half naked girls whom they cannot touch. But you should be able to answer that yourself by now; men enjoy watching naked women simply because they like naked women more than women with clothes on.

Remember you are here for your man's benefit, so enjoy whatever is on offer even if is not quite to your taste. A well-mannered lady can do no less. It is the very best of manners to behave properly in any given set of circumstances, and being relaxed and interested is what is required here.

In my experience the girls are happy to chat, and more than happy to chat with a woman and be complimented on their dancing. If you get the chance to have a word, take it. In many places the girls make most of their money from tips, but you will figure that out. Even when naked they will have a garter or something to tuck money in so give them a tip – you, not your man – and don't be mean. You are here to have fun as well as to impress him.

Get your man to buy you a lap dance if you can. The girl will come and dance just for you, usually between your knees as you sit on your chair. She will not touch you, and you are not meant to touch her, but do talk to her and compliment her on her beauty and her dancing. You will find that having a near naked body inches from you is an exciting experience. Her scent and her smooth, warm body swaying between your legs will be attractive even though you are probably not at all lesbian and would never dream of taking her to bed. It is good to tell her (and your man) that you find her sexy. Make your man give her a tip as a thank you.

By going to a girly bar you have at least accumulated an experience to discuss with your friends. I am sure they'll be jealous and you may find yourself escorting them for a return visit. You will also have made a significant impression on your man, who will certainly be seeing you through new and appreciative eyes.

Sex Shops
Sex shops vary a lot in quality, but the general standard is improving now that professional retail chains have been formed. They used to be hidden away in low rent areas, areas you probably would never visit, but now they are moving towards the town center. Most of them offer sex toys, lingerie, magazines and movies in a clean and brightly lit room. They do not seem very relaxing or even very naughty – apart from the fact that most of what they sell is designed to make you have ecstatic orgasms whether you want them or not.

Visiting sex shops with your man is fun. Everyone likes window-shopping, and this is window-shopping that you and your man can enjoy together. You may not have tried it before, probably out of embarrassment, and if that is true you have been a bad girl. You should not have deprived him of the pleasure of taking you around. In fact the embarrassment is all on your side. The other customers are not interested in you, and the sales people have seen it all before. And in the meantime, you've been denying your man the chance of doing something naughty with you.

Most sex shops sell very revealing lingerie but it is often overpriced. They tend to have a lot of stretch one-size-fits-all garments like body stockings, which come in sealed packets and have to be bought on trust. The bras and panties seem to owe more to imagination than comfort but you may find something that is exciting and comfortable. The best shops will have some good quality flimsy clothes that you can wear around the house and display yourself tastefully to your man (and the fantasy hunk who comes to clean your pool, fix the air conditioner etc.) You are more likely to find a fitting room in this sort of shop and I can guarantee you will not find it difficult to get him in to help. The only word of caution about these sexy clothes is, having bought them, don't forget to wear them! It really is not too much trouble to drop your normal clothes off before you relax in the evening and slip on something provocative. It shows you are thinking of him.

All sex shops will have a range of toys and these can be great fun for both of you. We will not go into detail about toys now because we will want to play with them later, but you can have a good look around, see what looks exciting, discuss the impossible dimensions of some of the larger ones and get his reaction to the plastic pussies and inflatable dolls. It's good fun (and it feels very naughty) to carry a glossy vibrator up to the man behind the counter when you both know that the toy he is wrapping will soon be nosing its way into your pussy and scrambling your brain. I don't think I could work in a shop like that; I'd be a nervous wreck after the first day of thinking about all the sexual activity I would not be getting a share of.

The magazine rack will hold magazines you have probably not seen before. They are often devoted to sexual specialties like anal sex or enormous breasts, and are of poor quality and have mind-numbing writing. You will notice that there are a great many magazines for gay men. This is probably because a gay couple has two male sex maniacs in it, where yours has only one. For my advice you are better off with the mainstream girly magazines because they are more professional and better presented.

Some sex shops also have a peep show facility in the back (complain to the city fathers if they don't). The best peep shows consist of a show room surrounded by discrete booths with time-operated windows. (The second best shows are actually video booths with a range of time-metered X-rated films.) The idea is that you pay for a period – say 15 minutes – in your booth, the window opens and you can watch the actress in the show room doing whatever is permitted in your area. This can be as basic as the sort of partial strip show you saw in the girly bar right through to real sex with a partner. Ask the sales person exactly what is on offer before you pay. You may have to smile at him to let the pair of you share the same booth; tell him it is your first time and you are frightened. It can be a fun thing to do on a Saturday afternoon and rates fairly highly on the scale of naughtiness.

Tripping Around

Cars play a large part in our sexual development. Many a virginity has been given up on a car back seat and drive-in movie theatres would not be half as popular if young folk could make love at home. Now you are a bit older, the car still offers possibilities.

I am now about to suggest something that most people have done at one time or another, and that you should have kept on doing long after the necessity for it had gone. Reach over to your man's lap as he works his way through the traffic and stroke his cock. Yes, yes, I know, it's dangerous, responsible people would never do something like that, he might crash and kill you both. I don't believe it. If taxi drivers can answer the radio and take all sorts of complicated instructions while weaving their way through heavy city traffic, then rest assured that your man can steer the car down quiet suburban streets with your little hand rubbing up and down between his legs.

It is very pleasant for him to have this low level of stimulation as he drives on. You will soon have a nice firm swelling under your fingers as he shows his appreciation. Unless you are driving in crowded city lanes in broad daylight, you can undo his zip and pull your little friend out of his hiding place. No one in the other cars can see what you are doing; in fact they might be doing just the same and you would never know. Drift your hand slowly up and down his shaft, just enough to keep him excited, but not enough to cause a crisis. If no one is watching and there is no police car on your tail, you might try a small lick, just as a hors d'oeuvre before the main meal later. Wait for a traffic signal if you are worried about driving him mad, but I am sure he will like it. Lots of people carry this right through to orgasm and apparently no one crashes the car. I suppose we would see a stream of men turning up in hospital accident departments with teeth marks on their equipment if crashing was at all common. But it's better that you don't go too far this time; keep it for another day.

After you've played with him for a while, try driving him nuts by playing with yourself as well. He loves looking at your pussy, and will love watching you play with it even more. Once, when I was younger and wiser, I admit I did this for my boyfriend. I slipped off my panties, and leaning back against the car door, lifted one leg onto the seat between us. After playing and displaying for a while, I pulled a banana out of the shopping and used it as an improvised dildo. What an experience! I can still taste the banana – we peeled it and shared the bruised fruit afterwards. (Now I'm feeling embarrassed.)

You don't think you could show your pussy off to him like that? Why ever not? If you can't show it to him, who can you show it to? You let your gynaecologist look at it, even probe and poke it, and stick brutal instruments inside you. Are you seriously ready to let a stranger do things like that to your treasured pussy but not let the one person who really cares about you see it?

It's a very big turn-on for him to be allowed to see up your skirt, and it is a cosmic erotic event for him to see you caressing and teasing your pussy into excitement. Men find watching a woman masturbate is very, very stimulating. The makers of blue movies know this and a masturbation scene is almost mandatory in their productions. So what's making you shy? If you look at your hang-ups you'll find that they are all excuses and that deep down there is no hard reason behind them. Except that you might not enjoy it, and there I can set your mind at rest. Once you have started, you will find it can be a very spicy experience, and knowing that he is watching will add considerably to your enjoyment.

Where are you driving in your car? Not straight home yet. Do you have a local beauty spot you can visit? Preferably choose one without too many people. Park overlooking the river or the sea, and jump out of the car quickly – you don't want him to grab you yet. Keep your knees together – he's only allowed to look at you when he can't do anything about it. If there is no one around, try sitting back against the hood of your car, hand in hand, and look at the view. Once he is settled, reach for his cock again and tease him some more. Think how pleasant it will be for both of you when you stroke him gently and point his erection out across the landscape (or seascape). If there are too many people around, take a bit of a walk until you can find a little privacy. Not too much, of course, you want to live a bit dangerously, don't you? It will be fun having to hug and kiss him to hide his rampant cock while the good citizens of your town walk their dogs behind you.

Bringing Him Home

Perhaps it is time to relent and take him home. You have teased and stimulated him for long enough and he is ready for the next act. Now you know what a terrorist feels like driving a car bomb into town. Apparently they also drive around with their bomb beside them, ticking and ready to explode. I hope you can get home first.

- 7 -

The anatomy of the clitoris was described in 1559 by Renaldus Columbus of Padua, who claimed that previous anatomists had overlooked the very existence of 'so pretty a thing'.
Leslet A Hall

We cannot, by an effort of the will, either command or restrain the erection of the penis; and yet it is evidently owing to the mind for sudden fear, or anything which fixes our attention strongly and all at once, makes this member quickly subside, though it were ever so fully erected.
Robert Whytt 1751

Basic Skills

How are your basic skills? Can you hold your head up at a dinner party and say honestly 'I know how to give a good blow job' or 'I always have half a dozen orgasms before I let my man come'? These are things that a well-educated lady should know about, just as she should know how to lay a formal table or serve red wine. I know that you did not learn about them at school, but you did not necessarily pick up the information as an adult either. It depends very much on who you practiced with, and probably how many of them as well.

Let's just run down a short check list of basic knowledge

Where is Everything?

I read on the internet of a recent survey in which less than 10% of American men managed to identify the clitoris on a diagram of a woman's pussy. That is a terrible state of affairs. Hasn't any woman taken these ignorant people in hand and shown them where everything is? Do they manage to pleasure their women by pure luck, or have they given up trying? Who knows?

Much more frightening is the large percentage of women who are very vague about their own geography. So, just to prove to yourself that you know what you are doing, get out a little mirror, sit on your bed and have a good look.

With your legs only partly open, your pussy is closed. As you have already cleaned away all the surplus hair from your lips, you can clearly see the plump outer lips that define your sex. These are the soft cushions that run from your mons to the back of your vagina, ending at the smooth, flat area in front of your anus called the perineum. Your outer lips are fun for your man to play with, and it feels nice when he squeezes them with his whole hand. They are not very sensitive of themselves but serve to protect the really delicate surfaces inside.

Your outer lips might be full and closed, covering everything inside, or they might be relatively smaller and allow your inner lips to burst out and protrude beyond them. As we said before, pussies have their own unique features, like faces. It doesn't matter what sort of outer and inner lips you have. All of them look nice to a man and the pleasure you experience is the same either way. (Of course, ladies with hidden inner lips complain that prominent ones look sexier, and those with exposed inner lips would love to have the smooth, hidden look. We can be funny like that.)

If you run your finger tip from your mons down into the furrow between your outer lips you will start to feel the shaft of your clitoris (or clit for short). Your clit is a magic little organ, capable of giving you an ocean of pleasure, more than you could ever handle. It is one of life's mysteries as to why such an important thing should be so small and hidden, but that is how it is. Actually, it has considerable roots extending into your body, but the bit you can feel under its protective hood seems to be about the length of a matchstick and a bit fatter. Its internal structure is similar to a penis and it does swell and harden when you are excited. If you want to take a good look at it, you will have to use your mirror and pull the hood back. Emerging from hiding you will find a little pink pearl, much smaller than a pea. (There is a small percentage women who are blessed with a much larger clit, more the size of your little finger, which can protrude in erection. Apparently – and who really knows? – having a big clit doesn't mean you get more enjoyment from it. It might mean your man can find it more easily and I should imagine it would be a pleasant thing for him to suck on, so if you are made this way I think I would say lucky girl!)

Note that the hood over your clit is very like a man's foreskin and moving it up and down is stimulating. Some women masturbate this way, and everyone enjoys having it done to them at least some of the time.

Your inner lips spring from the base of your clit – they are actually attached to it – and run to the back of your vaginal opening. They are very varied in shape and size and even in colour. A black girl's inner lips can be dark black, which is understandable. A very white blonde girl's lips can range from quite dark gray-brown to rosy pink through to pale pink or white. When you are not excited, your inner lips are normally wrinkled and twisted against each other. They do swell a little as you get heated up, and can be quite firm and rubbery when you are seriously excited.

Your vaginal entrance is at the back of your sex. If you (or your man) run a finger down between your lips, you will first feel the length of your clit, slide between your inner lips, over your urethral opening (where you pee from) and then fall into your vagina. If you skip over that moist, pink tunnel you will find your anus a couple of inches further back.

Your vagina is also remarkable. If you have ever watched a blue movie, you have probably been surprised at the way the girls accept enormous cocks and apparently enjoy having them pump vigorously in and out. If you think about it, even a normal sized cock pushed into you reaches most of the way to your navel, but you still let them in with pleasure. Of course, practice helps. With experience you can enjoy squatting over your man, something that you were probably uncomfortable with when you first started making love. Small-framed Asian girls continue to surprise big Western men by bouncing up and down on top of them and enjoying themselves on cocks that must be reaching far up into their tummies.

Perhaps more surprising than the length of cock you can accommodate is the width. Here the limit seems to be your bone structure. If you have wide hips you can accommodate more, but as a general rule a lady can happily accept a hand the size of her own in her vagina. That's right, your hand – your pussy. Remarkable, isn't it?

As a well educated lady, I'm sure the little geographical excursion above was not necessary but, still holding your mirror, I want you to try and imagine the problems your secret places pose for your man. When he first touched you he did not have the benefit of a road map. Do you remember when you first felt his fingers down there? I'm sure he could not see what he was doing. It was probably dark, and it's a good bet that you still had your panties on. Do you think you could have found your way around some-one else's pussy in those circumstances? Believe me, it's not easy to do with precision, and to add to the difficulty, every pussy likes to be stroked a different way. There is no approved method for playing with a pussy. What is good for one might drive another pussy owner insane. Or worse still, leave her cold and frustrated.

It is important that you realize how physically difficult you are to please. A man is guided by what he has been shown before, and if you are lucky he will have had open and intelligent lovers in the past. If not, you will have to educate him yourself if you and he are to have the experiences you both want.

How Good is your Pussy?

Relax; they're all good, including yours. Especially now you have started taking a little more care of it. The biggest complaint that most women have (apart from never being satisfied with its appearance) concerns lubrication. Don't worry; you're not alone. When your man first reached into your panties you were deliciously wet and slippery. Now you can still get wet, but it takes time and you never seem to get quite so juicy. That's life, I'm afraid. It happens to everyone, even the wettest and juiciest of us. I'm sure you still manage a presentable wetness when something unusual is happening to you, like making love in the alley behind the restaurant or when you just know the sexy young couple next door are peeping through the gap in your curtains. For the rest of the time, you will just have to do what everyone does and hit the bottle. It is a well-known fact that most of the women who buy baby oil in the supermarket don't have babies. As long as you enjoy the result, who cares?

The other complaint is 'I'm too loose...' I am no doctor and this is not a medical text, but now you are touching on something important. It is quite possible for women to lose muscle tone around their vaginas as they age, if they are not careful. Women who have had children may be more likely to suffer from this, and it can be a real problem as you get old. For the sake of your health it is important that you keep these muscles in good shape.

Note that I say 'for the sake of your health'; strong muscles are not absolutely necessary for good lovemaking. Having said that, there are women who take the muscles in their pussy seriously, and the results can be very pleasing for them and their men. A real courtesan should be able to 'milk' her man with her pussy, all without moving her hips. She can move his cock from side to side in her vagina. You can imagine that the chance to make love to a woman with a pussy like this has always been highly valued by men. This is what the Karma Sutra says about vaginal muscle control and the woman who has it. 'She must always lay stress on closing and constricting the Yoni (the vagina) until it holds the Lingam (the penis) as with a fist, opening and shutting at her pleasure, and finally acting as the hand of the Gopala-girl who milks the cow. This can be learned only by long practice, and especially by throwing the will into the part affected. Her husband will then value her above all women, nor would he exchange her for the most beautiful queen in the Three Worlds...'

Even if you just know that the most beautiful queen in the Three Worlds would not stand a chance with your man, still it would be nice to milk him like a Gopala-girl. Or if you can't manage that, to just hold him tight and squeeze him when you want to. Doctors prescribe exercises (Kegel exercises – look for them on the internet) that strengthen your muscles and give you the ability to squeeze if not to milk. They also give you better sensations and easier orgasms. The exercises are well known, but still the Western world is not full of Gopala-girls. That is because, like most forms of pure exercise, they are boring. They are also difficult to do correctly, which only adds to the problem.

There are exercise gadgets available that help you squeeze but they look as if they were designed by NASA; I would be cautious about letting one of these machines near my pussy. As a much more interesting alternative, try visiting www.jadeeggs.com. This company sells beautiful jade eggs in three different sizes. They are smooth and warm up quickly in your hand. The idea is to slip one into your pussy and hold it. If your muscles are weak, you will have trouble holding one of the larger ones inside. Never mind; as you squeeze and struggle to stop it slipping out, you are already exercising those important muscles. As you get stronger, you will be able to hold smaller and smaller eggs, and hold them for longer periods. They are perfectly hygienic and safe; they even look pretty. And they cannot get lost inside because there is nowhere for them to go. If one is being awkward and refusing to come back out into the cold, you just squat and lay the egg – like a chicken.

As an expert you can do two things with the eggs. Firstly, some have a small hole drilled right through them. You can put a thread through one and use it to hang weights on. The company recommends that you do not start with more than 10 pounds weight unless you are already an expert. 10 pounds! Can you imagine being able to hold 10 pounds just by squeezing your pussy muscles? Actually, it's not as difficult as it sounds, provided that you have done some practicing first. And if that is what you can do, what do the so-called experts manage to support? I can't imagine – but I do know a pussy like that would interest any man.

The most advanced thing you can do with your eggs is to insert two small ones and then use all the different muscles around your vagina to move them around inside you, even tap them together. This is much more difficult but you will feel a sense of achievement when you first get them to move around. You will be proud of yourself, and I am absolutely sure that your man will feel the same way when he thinks of you exercising your pussy to provide him with the ultimate sheath for his sword. Move over, Gopala-girl!

Of Course I know what a Penis looks like!

Yes, yes, I'm sure you do. Every girl has played with at least a few of them in her unmentionable past. Excuse me being doubtful, but let's just quickly run over a few points in case there is something you have missed. Cocks are as variable as pussies and each has its own personality. They can be long, thin, short, fat, you name it. Few of them are absolutely straight and some have quite alarming bends in them; it all adds to the fun. Whatever their appearance, there are a few things they have in common that you should be completely familiar with.

Firstly, and this is especially true in the States, cocks come in two types – circumcised and uncircumcised. Also known as cut and uncut or natural. As an aside, there are three main bodies of opinion that support circumcision; the Muslim faith, the Jewish faith and the AMA. I know about the motives of the first two, but I am not going to speculate on the motives of the third. I might get sued. (For what my opinion is worth, I don't have any time for the religious motives either. If the Good Lord creates male babies with foreskins, who are the sex-obsessed old men to insist that He made a mistake that must be corrected by cutting it off. If you have a son, at least let him make up his own mind when he is old enough.)

Sorry, enough sexual politics. We'll get back to the fact that you will have either one sort or the other to play with. The consensus is that when they are inside you, it is hard to feel any difference. During oral sex, you will be pulling the foreskin back anyway, so your technique and its effects are identical. When you play with a natural cock by hand or in other ways – say between your breasts – you will find that the foreskin can be moved up and down over the glans (or head). This is very stimulating and he will enjoy it. For a while, this sliding back and forth doesn't need any lubrication. As you continue he may contribute some himself (a clear, slippery liquid like your own), or you can give him a quick lick to moisten him. Without a foreskin, a cut penis has to be stimulated by stroking the glans directly with your hand, so lubrication is a little more critical. Of course, he will still contribute but without a foreskin to retain moisture, the glans seems to dry out more quickly.

The glans is where it all happens. I guess you can think of the concentration of nerve endings there as similar to your clit. Only a similar number of nerve endings – bigger doesn't mean men get more of those delightful endings. The main difference is that men are not blessed with all the other very pleasurable areas you have between your lips and into your vagina. Poor men! Still, having all the sensitive points concentrated somewhere so obvious does make your job a lot easier. The whole glans is sensitive. It likes being stroked, squeezed, licked, breathed on, rubbed with ice, you name it, the glans will respond happily. Do anything to it rhythmically and for long enough and you will induce an orgasm. But if you can't go wrong with the glans, you can always do better. You will find the most sensitive place is just under the rim of the head, where it joins onto the skin of the shaft. Pulling back firmly on the skin covering of the shaft puts a delightful tension on this join and we will discuss later how you can use this tension to refine the pleasure you give your man.

Most of his cock is made up of the shaft and here I suppose we ought to talk about size. For some reason men are sensitive about the size of their cocks, and this is especially true of American men. It doesn't matter that women say any cock of a more or less normal size is satisfactory, and that anyway technique is far more important than length, still men worry about size. If only they put half as much effort into worrying about their partner's body! Anyway, I know you are not going to trade in your man for the hope of getting one with a bigger cock, so just be careful to caress away any feeling of inadequacy. Try to express delight at its size now and again, and assure him that it really is the most handsome and satisfactory one you have ever experienced. In this area a few white lies and a little flattery will get you a long way.

The shaft of his cock and his balls are not particularly sensitive, in the sense that handling them will not make him come. However it does feel very nice to have a lady's hand manipulating and stroking them, and your man will allow you to hold him whenever you like. Men are very generous in that way.

I am sure that you do not need to be told that his balls are delicate and you can hurt him dreadfully just by being too enthusiastic with them. Many of your sisters (not you, I'm sure) just do not seem to know what to do with their boyfriend's balls. Please study the following carefully so you will be able to instruct them. A man's balls are held in a sac, known as the scrotum or more commonly as the bag. This bag looks simple enough but seems to have a mind of its own. At rest it is loose and stretched out. The balls hang low and swing as he moves. In cold weather it wrinkles up into a firm, furry pouch and the balls are held tightly under the base of his shaft. Sexual stimulation has the same effect and this is how they will usually appear when you are playing with him and he is excited.

It is very pleasant for him when you hold his balls in your cupped hand and gently move the whole bag around. Or brush backwards and forwards across its surface with the side of a finger or thumb. It is not the sort of intense pleasure you would give him by doing the same thing to his glans, nor is there the same slow pain/pleasure transition that you can give him by squeezing his glans or dragging your teeth across it. He also loves you kissing him there, brushing him with your hair and breathing on him. Having you manipulate his balls individually is interesting, but the slightest over-pressure is immediately agonizing. You must keep your caresses gentle even when you are getting excited over oral sex. In fact, especially during oral sex, when an inadvertent squeeze could result in you getting choked.

Finally, and usually neglected by women, is the strip of smooth skin between the back of his balls and his anus. A female fingertip gently brushing or scratching backwards and forwards in this area is very stimulating. And a wet tongue is even better.

- 8 -

*A dress makes no sense unless it inspires men
to want to take it off you.*
Françoise Sagan

GARTHER, *n. An elastic band intended to keep a woman from coming out
of her stockings and desolating the country.*
Ambrose Bierce The Devil's Dictionary

Keeping the Pot Boiling

So where did we leave you and your man? As I recall you were taking the scenic route home, and you had pulled his cock out and were pointing it at the car roof. Massaging him gently to keep his interest, but not enough to distract him from driving. Very good; you have one hundred percent of his attention for the moment, but what are you going to do when you get home?

You don't want to rush straight off to the bedroom as soon as the front door closes behind you. Not today, anyway. There is a lot to be said for an emergency quickie up against the wall – Erica Jong's famous zipless fuck. Spontaneity and quick release are good for both of you sometimes, but today we are looking for something longer and more refined.

You will need to get him comfortable and waiting for you with his tongue hanging out, while you get ready for the next act. At minimum you are going to need a quick change of clothes. And you are going to need nibbles and drinks if you are going to make an evening of it.

The Blessings of Pornography

Pornography – or erotica if you are insisting on being highbrow – is a lot more fun and a lot more available than it used to be. The internet was designed as a pure tool for private communication between human beings and, because they are human beings, it was immediately used for the most important thing in life – sex. A staggering percentage of internet traffic is pornography; I have read estimates as high as 80%. This is not surprising; the earliest statuettes from the dawn of human prehistory were of buxom, naked women so you could say it is in our blood. I have heard (but don't quote me) that one of the very first photographs was of a young lady entertaining a Shetland pony in a Parisian studio. And so the internet is inevitably seen as a private gateway to an Aladdin's cave of porn – a pornucopia, in fact.

A wide range of material and sensations are on offer. Some of it is of the highest quality and would try the resolve of the most determined saint. On the other hand, a lot of it is excruciatingly bad and some of it is outright illegal even in the most liberal of countries. Its only drawback from your point of view is that it tends to be a rather solitary opportunity. That is no reason not to spend an evening seated on your man's lap surfing the ocean of sexy material out there. In fact now download speeds are so much faster, many couples are buying online video cams and sharing live sex with like-minded lovers. Good for them!

However, tonight you want to be the centre of his attention so leave the computer switched off and provide him with a magazine you thoughtfully purchased in advance. This will give you time to disappear, get changed, break out the biscuits and dip, uncork the wine.

Try and buy a magazine that you will find stimulating too. I would suggest one of the better class ones like Penthouse or perhaps Hustler. Not Playboy; it takes itself too seriously and any girly magazine that can include interviews with US presidents is nothing like naughty enough. At the other end of the scale are the magazines for the semi-literate that are mostly ads and photos. Now I know you are both literate and well educated (or you wouldn't be enjoying this book) so you will need something with more interesting writing and well-shot, erotic photographs. I have a copy of Penthouse in front of me at the moment; it has articles on the Cold War military, a man walking around the world, anti-semitism and Kenny Chesney the country star. Getting a little more sexy there are articles on women who cheat, interracial wife swapping and the regular forums. Hotter still there are readers' letters and Xaviera Hollander writing her own brand of advice.

And finally the photos, just four sets of first quality portraits. One of these is of a wholesome young American girl getting to know the pizza delivery boy very, very intimately (and deeply). Unusually there are two 'lesbian' sequences, one with the bizarrely dressed Catwoman and the other in artistic black-and-white. (Normally there would be only one girl-on-girl set. Why are straight men so interested in the idea of lesbians? Real lesbians make it quite clear that they have no use for men and certainly do not want them watching as they make love. I suspect the main reason that men prefer seeing a lesbian couple over a straight couple is that the lesbian one has twice as many pussies! Just my theory.) The central photographic sequence is of a beautiful woman Lily Ann, beautifully presented by the famous Suze Randall, one of the best glamour photographers in the business and, incidentally, a woman.

There! Nothing that will make you squirm with embarrassment at the newsagents, and you should even be able to share your man's appreciation by reading it together. And I can guarantee that giving him a naughty present like Penthouse will make him think he's got a girl in a million.

Would a sexy DVD do instead of a magazine? I wouldn't recommend it. Anything on DVD tends to be much more stimulating and demanding of his attention. Keep the DVDs for the evenings when you want to share a little hot theatre together.

Once you've got him settled with a kiss, a squeeze and his magazine, rush to get him a drink. Men appreciate something to suck on while they're concentrating. You can now take off and get changed. Changed into what? Well, it has to look provocative of course. And it has to be practical, by which I mean it has to keep you warm enough (it's difficult to enjoy lovemaking when you're turning blue with cold) and it has to allow easy access to your sexy bits. So avoid anything with too many hooks and eyes. A revealing bra might be acceptable but a full bra – no matter how pretty – is out of the question. Likewise, be cautious about clothes that have to be removed over your head; wrestling with those can be a killer. Things that push down over your hips are OK; he can do that without breaking a kiss. You are really looking for something that opens at the front so he can reach your most interesting features without completely undressing you (yet).

Conventional pantyhose are out because they are all covering and are difficult to take off when engaged at close quarters. The exotic tights that are made like stockings and garter belt are a possibility. Men are strange about stockings. It used to be thought they loved them so much because when they were youngsters their first girl friends wore stockings and so they became fixated on stockinged legs. That theory has been disproved because a whole generation or more of men has grown up never knowing stockings worn in earnest, and still they are popular. Stockings are inconvenient and the suspenders are uncomfortable. They even limit the shortness of your skirts and so you would expect men to complain. But the truth is that stockings have one overwhelming and delightful advantage; he can remove your panties without taking the stockings off. Providing you have remembered to put them on last, of course. And a woman wearing stockings and a garter belt is displaying her pussy and her bottom in the same way that the picture frame displays the Mona Lisa. Really – believe me! Every lady should have old-fashioned stockings and garter belt in her panty drawer for occasions like tonight. Nowadays they are worn exclusively for making love and when you see how much your man enjoys making love to you in stockings, you will start liking them too – never mind the inconvenience.

As for the rest, I can only echo the cry of Government reformers everywhere – transparency is the fundamental requirement. Your clothes can cover you, just as long as they don't hide you. Don't leave off your jewellery and make-up; if you wear them for going out, you should certainly wear them for your man. You can even wear those impossibly uncomfortable high heels – it's not far to walk before you collapse on top of him.

Laying down the Law

Tonight is the night when you are going to be calling the shots and your man will just have to sit still and be your sex object. It will clear up any confusion if you get his agreement right from the start. He might find it a little strange, but he'll soon take to the idea, trust me.

It's Showtime!

So you come trotting out of the kitchen with the drinks and nibbles, wearing clothes that scream 'Take me! Now!' He's sitting on the sofa, soft music is playing, and he's drooling in anticipation of the nice things that are going to be served up for his pleasure. Do you want him to change as well, or are you going to enjoy taking off his normal clothes? Up to you, but if you want him to slip into that short Chinese silk dressing gown you bought him for Christmas, now is a good time to do it. It won't take long, believe me.

How will you start the ball rolling? You're the boss, so you get to decide. Try going around the back of the sofa where he can't reach you. Massage his shoulders and run your hands down his front to brush against his cock. Kiss him as you tease it; doing both at once is irresistible. Stand out of reach and pose for him. Give him a lap dance, with no touching of course. I wouldn't be in a hurry to do a strip tease for him – there will be plenty of time to get out of your clothes later. You can offer him the chance to take off your panties, but insist on him doing this with his teeth. The best way to do this is... but why should I tell you and spoil the fun of finding out for yourself? Just be careful not to let the sofa tip over backwards.

Keep on Teasing

Classically, serious lovemaking starts with the woman teasing the man into activity and then moves to the man using all his skill to build up the woman's excitement to unbearable levels and beyond. The final act is when his cock is inside you, being stimulated to the climax that brings your little piece of theatre to an end.

Start by kissing and stroking him, but play with his cock right from the start. If the tables were turned you would probably prefer a long period of kissing and caressing before he reaches your pussy, but that is because you are a woman. Men need a more direct approach. They still enjoy being kissed and caressed, but they prefer you to be holding their cock while you do it.

Try getting him onto his back on the floor. If you don't have the classical bearskin rug to make love on, throw down a duvet or a blanket. It is good to make love on a firm surface; you will be able to bounce up and down on top of him with much more precision. You can also give him an erotic dance – he's never watched you dancing from this angle. Lying on the floor and looking up your long legs to where your panties used to be will give him something to remember.

As you are dancing, get closer and closer to him until you are on all fours and he is completely under your shadow. To start touching him, try approaching from the head and kissing him upside down – it makes a change and you can still reach his cock comfortably. He will love the feeling of being inside the tent of your hair and clothes, and you can drive him mad by trailing your breasts over his face and chest. Try and keep him away from your pussy; for the moment you want to keep a clear head.

If you wish you can allow the sexual excitement of lovemaking to build in a smooth crescendo, ratcheting up the tension and allowing yourself no more than the smallest of orgasms, until you reach the final (and hopefully mutual) explosion. This is great fun but difficult to do successfully. It is even more difficult to achieve if you want to stretch your lovemaking session out to an hour or more. In practice you will find yourself following the alternative route more often – building up to a plateau and enjoying gently rising and falling levels of excitement until he has given you enough orgasms and you are ready to enjoy his.

Your man's physiology lends itself readily to this second approach. As you play with his cock the pressure will build up to a point where he can come with very little extra stimulation. If stimulation is withdrawn at this moment or slowed right down, he will become less sensitive and instead of the pot boiling over, it stays at a comfortable simmer. It is this plateau of excitement that you need to control if you are going to give your man the extended pleasure he is capable of. Wise lovers deliberately slow down and keep him within a minute or two of orgasm for as long as they can.

The good news is that it is not very difficult to keep your man in a state of semi-ecstasy. You probably know already the signs of his impending orgasm (I hope you have at least studied that much very carefully) so when you read them, slow down or even stop. Avoid his glans for a moment or two and when you return to it, be gentle. If his cock starts to show any sign of softness, speed up your efforts for a few moments until it is satisfactorily rigid again. By craft and cunning you should be able to keep him on edge for hours.

Offer him Candy

The tastiest thing around will be sexy, juicy you, so be generous and let him enjoy as much of you as possible. Rub your whole body over him. Lie on top of him and smother him with your softness. Don't worry about squashing him. He's tough and well able to support your weight as you wriggle over him. Try kneeling above his head and holding his wrists to the floor by his sides. In this position you are free to use your breasts and your long hair on his chest and face, besides reaching far enough down his body to give his cock an occasional lick. Let him feast on your breasts and torment your nipples. Give his nipples extra attention; they might not be as sensitive as yours, but he'll still enjoy your efforts.

Don't forget his back. Roll him over and rub yourself over his butt and his back. When you position him this way up, make sure you pull his cock down so it is pointing towards his feet. This is not as uncomfortable as it looks, and it is much better than having it trapped beneath his tummy. You can now play gently with it as you trail your hair over his shoulders, back and butt.

Besides your breasts, use your pussy. Let him look at it, of course, and kiss him with it, all over his body. Big, slippery, wet kisses – he'll be in heaven. He will enjoy seeing your pussy smiling while you kneel over him. He will probably bury his face in it if you are not careful to stay out of range, but try and keep him under control. Kneel around his head and press your pussy onto his forehead while you stroke his body and play with his cock. Imagine how provoking that will feel to him; your hot, wet pussy pressing his head to the floor, out of sight, out of reach and infinitely desirable.

Time out

Take time out to sip your drinks, nibble and chat. Talk about sex, about the things you're going to do to him when you've finished your glass of wine. If he responds to dirty talk, now is a good time to use it. Accuse him of ogling other women and tell him you know what was going through his mind as he watched them. Tell him you're going to punish him with teeth marks on his cock.

Don't be concerned if his cock starts to relax; you'll soon have it standing tall again.

About this time you should really make a judgment about whether your man is going to stay the course, or if you have got him so hot and excited that he is ready to explode at the slightest bit of over-enthusiasm on your part. This is very important to a subtle, scheming lover (as you are this evening) because if your man is uncontrollable, you will need to do something to relieve the pressure. If he is too much on edge, the best thing is a quick orgasm, early on; the alternative is to change your game plan and accept that you have been too successful in turning him on and a long, languid lovemaking session is off the menu for tonight.

Question : when do men want to come twice? Answer : before they've come once. It's true; no matter how hungry and excited he is before he comes, he will experience a great sense of relaxation when you give him his first orgasm. And the more tension you've built up, the longer you've taken up to this point, the bigger the orgasm and relaxation will be. But don't worry about it; he just needs a ten-minute break. You can hold his cock during this time, but don't try to stimulate it yet. Take the opportunity of another time out, a chat, drink, perhaps a nibble, and then you can start working on his cock. You'll soon have the show back on the road again.

Tantalize

I hope by now that you are completely convinced that as well as loving you, he loves your body. There is nothing you can do (apart from getting up to wash the dishes or do the ironing) that will stop him wanting to eat you up. All you can hope to do is delay that happy event, and the longer you hold him back, the more you will both enjoy it in the end. Try offering your opulent body to him, but keep him where he can't reach it.

With him lying on his back, put his arms by his sides and kneel astride his tummy. In this position your knees and calves keep his arms pressed to his sides. He will feel trapped even though you both know he could throw you off in seconds. You will also be sitting on the head of his cock, lying flat on his stomach. (You are doing this not because it feels good for you and him but purely to keep him out of mischief; so no unauthorized wriggling is allowed. That comes later.)

He can see you very well so this is a good time to discuss your breasts with him. Hold them in your cupped hands, move them around, point them at him and extract as many compliments as you can. Don't hold back but openly play with them. Show him everything that feels good. Tease and squeeze your nipples and let him see how much you enjoy them. If you are one of the small band of happy girls who can come by just teasing their breasts, now is the time to show him your party piece. If you can't quite manage that, at least make sure he understands how excited you are becoming. If you know that you are naturally very quiet and not given to sexy sighs and moans, don't rely on him guessing your excitement from the glazed look in your eyes. Tell him straight out and move around enough so that he can appreciate how wet your pussy has become.

The man who doesn't enjoy the sight of a woman playing with her pussy has not yet been born, so swallow any remaining inhibitions and let him celebrate with you. Don't even think of being shy and holding back, or you'll have my disappointment to add to your own. Pop a small cushion under his head so that he can watch comfortably, tip your hips back and display his favorite pussy to him. It is a good idea to shuffle up to his chest so he can see more closely; just outside licking distance is about right. Touch and caress your pussy as you would like him to do it. Talk to him about it; make him beg you to show him more. Spread your lips apart and ask him if he can see your clit. Entice it out of its hiding place and do nice things to it. Dip a finger into your vagina and give it to him to lick – why not? His tongue will be way up inside you shortly and he will be wet from ear to ear, so why should you suddenly go all coy about giving him a wet finger to lick? For sure he will suck your finger like a calf if you give him the chance, and your generosity will give him a big buzz.

Reach as far inside you as you can, and tell him how good it feels. Ask him if he can see up inside you. Regardless of his answer pull your vagina open with a finger from each hand and watch his face as he stares into the darkness. Do nice things to your whole pussy but try to remember that you are showing off so keep on spreading and pulling your inner lips and displaying your clit. Finally, when you are getting too hot and confused yourself, give him one of your orgasms. Sharing this very intimate moment with him will make him realize how lucky he is to have you. It will scramble his brain as much as yours and it will be time for a short intermission.

Slowing Down Again

How are you going? Are you following the script so far? Do you think you could possibly invite him to look at you so closely, or even watch while you rub yourself to an orgasm? If your first reaction is 'Interesting – but I could never do that!', don't worry. 99% of your sisters have probably said the same thing at some time in their lives. Fortunately as girls get older and wiser, they generally start to feel more confident and less worried about what other people might say if they knew. Either that or they realize that no one other than their man will ever know, and you can take his vote for granted. He loves your pussy and he loves it even more when you are hot and excited. If you are still reluctant to give these little pleasures to your man, at least keep my suggestions in the back of your mind and, when you are crazy with sex, who knows what might happen?

I am serious about letting him watch your orgasms. Inviting him to watch something so secret is a great gesture of love for him. If you feel impossibly awkward about it, try asking him to show you as well

– I'll do mine if you do yours. This is really intimate and sophisticated sex, as you will find if you watch his eyes while it is happening.

Enough sexy thoughts for the moment, it's time to let him cool down a little. While you are taking a break, let's talk about a couple of skills that you should master – oral sex and the ultimate hand job. We'll consider them both as if you were going to carry them through to completion, although tonight you are just going to use them to pile on the pressure and get him ready for the final act.

- 9 -

Clinton lied. A man might forget where he parks or where he lives, but he never forgets oral sex, no matter how bad it is.
Barbara Bush (Former First Lady)

You're the one I want to forever please
Lick you, suck you, taste you and tease
Rhonda Forever Kind of Ecstasy

A Special Kind of Treat

Oral sex, or fellatio or giving head or a blow job if you prefer, is one of the most wonderful experiences you can offer your man. It is also one in which you have the strictest and most precise control of his ascent to orgasm and the intensity of the orgasm itself. So it is essential that you teach yourself how to draw the last drop of ecstasy from it before you can hold your head up at your next parent teacher meeting where you will be starring as the amateur courtesan who is rumoured to put the professionals in the shade.

Having said that, you will be aware that fellatio can be a very contentious issue, even political. Fundamentalist Christians are joined by rabid feminists in either rejecting - or at least feeling very uncomfortable with – the whole idea. Never mind; as Homer Simpson said, 'When the authorities warn you of the dangers of having sex, there is an important lesson to be learned. Do not have sex with the authorities.'

In fact, they are looking at it through very distorting lens. Although a woman on her knees in front of a man might appear servile, in fact she is definitely the boss. She has her hands on all the levers, and her man had better not forget it. After all, those are sharp white teeth wrapped around his cock and he should not take his woman for granted. She has total control over whether he gets lucky or not, and of the act itself. A man doesn't 'do oral sex' on a woman; he receives it – if he is a good boy and shows sufficient gratitude afterwards.

And it is not just a one-way experience. You are meant to enjoy it too. One of the great experiences in life is sucking his small, soft grape into your mouth and letting it rest there while it grows into a swollen and hungry plum. Or feeling him taut and trembling, and knowing that every slight and clever movement of your mouth and hands is strumming the stretched nerves of his soul. What a feeling of power!

Starting from Basics

The first thing you have to do is get comfortable. You may be sucking his cock for some time so take a position that suits you both. Perhaps the best way is to have him sit on the edge of the sofa so you can kneel between his legs and have both access and freedom of movement. You can also lay him on the floor and lean over him, but this can get tiring after a while as you support yourself with one arm. Putting him on all fours and lying on your back with your head between his knees can be good, but only if his cock is neither too long nor too short. Too long will pin you to the floor by the tonsils, and too short means that you can only get enough of him in your mouth by continually lifting your head – again too much of a strain.

You should avoid any position that gives him too much opportunity for movement if you are restricted. You don't want him to make an uncontrolled thrust as he comes unless you can move with it, so don't get between him and a chair back! He really doesn't need to move much during conventional fellatio as you are doing all that for him. A good compromise position is for both of you to lie on your sides, with a firm cushion under your head to lift your mouth up to the level of his cock. This way he can move a little, and you can relax your neck muscles.

However you position yourself, and whether you approach his cock from below, or above, or from the side, always remember that you can't give a superb blowjob without your hands. Your hands are at least 50% of the experience so one or preferably both of them must be free to help.

Look and Lick

Start by holding his cock and studying it carefully. Even if it is an old friend and has been inside you thousands of times, he will enjoy watching you explore it. Pull his foreskin back if he has one, and look at it from all angles. An experimental lick or two is in order, especially burrowing the tip of your tongue into spots under the rim of the glans. Kisses all over and down to his balls are also welcome. Then close your mouth, run your tongue over your lips to wet them, look him straight in the eye and suck the whole glans slowly into your mouth. Don't just open your mouth and pop it in; suck him in with a long slow slurp. You are now ready to start in earnest.

It is surprising how many ladies think that fellatio consists of bobbing their head up and down so that their lover's cock slips in and out of their mouth. While it is true that this feels good to your man, it doesn't feel as good as doing the same thing in your pussy which, after all, is designed to do just that. Neither is it essential to force his cock deep into your mouth. Again, your pussy specializes in that and does it better.

What your pussy can't do – and your mouth does extremely well – is lick and suck; roll your tongue up and torment the slit at the end; lick round and around the rim of the glans; flick-flick-flick at the web of skin between the two ribs on the lower side of the glans – in fact a whole galaxy of different sensations. All of these things are intensely exciting, and you can only give them to him with your mouth.

So suck it in and hold it in your warm mouth for a while. Explore it with your tongue. The texture is smooth and rubbery. Once in my student days I was sitting with a girl friend after an enjoyable meal in a Chinese restaurant. On her spoon she passed me one of the tinned lychees she was having for dessert. "That feels just like my boyfriend," she said. Mmmh.

You are holding his cock in your hand while you explore the glans, and if he has a foreskin you are holding it back so you can run your tongue around all those exciting corners. Foreskin or not, you should be holding the skin of his shaft back firmly. This pulls at the join between the glans and the shaft, and stretches those sensitive nerves endings. Stretched out like this they are at the mercy of your tongue tip as you flick it back and forth around the join. Keep watching him while you do this because if there is any sign he is getting too excited, you must back off quickly. Just relax the tension your hand is giving him, and leave the glans alone.

Men will let you lick and suck at the head of their cock for just as long as you like, and in fact many women complain that they don't like fellatio because it is tiring to keep their mouth open for so long. This is just an excuse for bad technique and shows that the women concerned don't really care. Of course keeping your mouth wide open for long periods is uncomfortable – who enjoys going to the dentist? So shut it! Keep his cock in your mouth as long as you are comfortable, and then take it out and do something else. Lick it. Give it big wet kisses and sucks using just your lips with your teeth closed. Hold his prick up and bury your face in his balls. Poke your tongue at the end of it and work with your hands for a while. Kiss his balls (gently) and nibble at his bag with your lips. He will enjoy all of those things.

In the first phase of your work try all sorts of caresses and, of course, repeat those that have the most interesting effect on him. At this point you do not need any sort of rhythm. That comes next.

Building up

Your mouth is wet and soft, and one of the delightful things you can do to him is to move him around inside it. With your mouth relaxed and open just enough to keep your teeth clear, put the glans or part of it in your mouth and move your head gently from side to side. Don't worry if you dribble a bit; it all adds to the luxurious feeling you will be giving him. If you wanted to, you could make him come just like this. It is such a relaxed method that you can even do it lying on your back with him resting his tip on (rather than in) your mouth from the side.

Although the most intense and enjoyable sensations come from your mouth, the drive to orgasm should ideally come from your hands. Cup his balls in one hand and gently brush and manipulate his bag. With the other hand, work the skin on his shaft back and forth.

As you are licking and sucking at his glans, the range of movement of your hand is necessarily limited so here is a technique that is guaranteed to drive him mad.

Pull the skin on his shaft back positively until it tugs at the glans. Then pull back harder until it is really tight – your man will let you know if you overdo this – and relax again but only far enough to reduce the tension, not so far that the tension disappears. Just go from tight to very tight and back again. And now repeat this stroke, slowly at first, faster as you approach his orgasm.

Remember that it is your hand that gives him the orgasm, not your mouth. Your hand makes the orgasm, and your mouth makes sure the orgasm is the most fantastic, intense and explosive experience possible. The combination of your mouth on his glans and your hand on the shaft is what will give him the perfect blow job.

The Twist

A small addition to your technique that will have him begging for more. As we described above, you are driving him wild by moving your hand from holding the skin tight to pulling it back firmly. To add a little spice, when you have the skin firmly back, increase the torment by giving the skin a quarter twist around the shaft. This twisting gives a sharp tweak to the pleasure he is receiving each time you do it. You might find it a little difficult to learn the movement well enough so that it becomes automatic. It's a bit like dancing; you can't really enjoy it until you don't have to think what your feet are doing. But it's certainly worth the effort to learn. Your hand makes three movements. From the starting position of holding the skin back with moderate tension, move down the shaft to increase the tension. Then twist around the shaft about a quarter turn to increase the tension to the limit. Then return to the starting position. It sounds easy enough, and so it is, but you need to have it down pat if you are to keep it up during the excitement of his orgasm.

The Big Event

As his excitement mounts, all his signals will be feeding back to you and you will naturally want to speed up and work harder for him. Resist the temptation! Not completely, of course, but the longer you spin out your efforts, the more rewarding the final explosion will be. Take him to the edge, and then stop with your hand and mouth relaxed. You will feel the pressure decline, and after a minute or so you can start again. Repeat this for as long as you like; the more times you almost let him come, the more spectacular it will be when he finally does. Volcanic is the word.

The Big Question

The big question, of course, is what do you do when he comes? Do you let him come in your mouth? Do you spit it out or swallow it? Do you let him come at all?

A lot of thought and energy has been expended on these questions. With the emancipation of women during the twentieth century, there was a growing feeling that no man – not even a husband – should have the power to force a woman into something that she doesn't want to do. This concept is now almost universally accepted. In theory a woman can say to her husband 'Get out of my pussy, I've changed my mind' when he is within a couple of strokes of orgasm, and she will have the full support of the law and society. I am sure that you will agree that this is not an agreeable or effective way for lovers to behave. We all have to think about what our partners want and whether we want to give it to them.

I suppose there are men who don't like to give their women the fun of oral sex, although I can't say I've ever met any (thank God!) Let us suppose such a man exists, what should be his attitude? Should he say my woman wants it so I must give it to her, or on the other hand can he say I don't like the idea so it's out of the question? Difficult, isn't it? The truth is, of course, that most of us live in the gray area in between. We don't particularly like something, or it's boring or difficult, but because our lover enjoys it we're prepared to go along. We enjoy our partner's pleasure, and are hopeful that our compliance will be rewarded by something nice in return.

No one is going to say that you must let him come in your mouth, but think about what exactly he is asking you to do. Even at his hungriest, he is only going to produce a teaspoon or so of come, so you are not going to drown. It doesn't taste completely revolting –

you've taken medicine that is far worse – and it's not going to poison you. So any uneasiness you might have is just about the idea of it. Some people won't eat prawns or avocado because they don't like the idea or the feel on their tongues (and that just makes them taste all the worse). If they can't enjoy prawns and avocado, it's their loss and there's more left for the rest of us, but if you can't give your lover a complete blow job, it's his loss as well as yours.

Most couples arrive at some sort of compromise. Some moral and very strong minded women actually refuse oral sex on themselves because they don't want to suck their men to completion – that really is a case of throwing the baby out with the bathwater. Many women seem to give their man some fun until he is ready to come, and then finish him off either by hand or with their pussy. Don't feel embarrassed if you are one of these. No one is being judgmental – except you yourself, of course.

If you are being self-critical, for once I have to agree with you. Imagine how he feels about it: you have been working hard at him, putting all your skill and heart into bringing on an agonizing, ecstatic orgasm, and at the last minute what are you going to do? You're going to take him out of your hot, wet, inviting mouth and point him at the ceiling? What sort of message does that send? He's your man and it's his come he's giving you. You can reject it, of course, but do you really want to? He doesn't particularly want you to swallow it, but he does want to be inside you when he comes. If you had a cock, wouldn't you feel the same?

Practically speaking it's difficult to refuse, so what are you going to do? One strategy is to make sure he is well back in your throat as he comes. A quick swallow, just like taking a pill, and the problem has gone. If you don't like to do that, just hold it in your mouth. Once he has finished, turn yourself around and share it with him in a big kiss. This is called snowballing and has the advantage of being very politically correct. Or you can just let it go, drop it on him or the bed sheet, where ever, and wipe your mouth with the corner of the sheet. Don't make a big deal of spitting it out; that's rude and bad manners.

It's also very rude to run to the bathroom and gargle mouthwash. This sort of behaviour is not lady-like so don't do it!

Now your wrist has been slapped, it's time for the good news. After you have done it a couple of times and realized that it's not so difficult, you will be free to enjoy the event. The feeling of him pulsing and spurting inside your mouth is so intimate it can't be matched. You will love it. And if you are not drowned in roses and chocolates in recognition of your new skills I shall be surprised.

Wheee!

You will feel his orgasm starting in his balls, in the hardness of his cock and in the tensing of all the muscles in his body. His come will spurt from him in great pulses. Try and meet it by squeezing his glans rapidly and rhythmically. This is a deliriously exciting moment for him, and pretty good for you too as you enjoy the orgasm that you created with your skilful mouth and hands.

Males are not as fortunate with their orgasms as females; when they come the event is very clearly defined and they cannot extend it into further moments of pleasure as we can. So if you can't make it longer, how can you make it better? Try this. Cover your teeth with your lips and take only half of his glans in your mouth. As he comes bite down hard on it a bit faster than once a second until he stops pulsing. Put an arm around him and hold on tight when you are doing this because he is likely to heave and thresh around in ecstasy and could easily throw you out of bed. If you have never done this to him before, keep it as a surprise; he will definitely be appreciative! You can have a similar but more gentle effect by sucking hard and rhythmically.

And the Golden Rule - whatever you are doing to him as he comes, don't stop until the last spurt.

Once he has come, he will be very sensitive so stop the stimulation dead and just hold suction on him until he is completely relaxed.

Why 69 doesn't Work

69 doesn't work for most people because receiving a good orgasm from oral sex is so mind-blowing that it's completely impossible to

do anything else at the same time. Playing with someone carefully at that instant just isn't an option. Sorry, but there it is.

69 is a good idea while you are starting off. While you are still coherent you can lick each other very enjoyably. It's fun to take turns, one person licking for a while and then relaxing to enjoy some licking in return. As you get hotter and hotter, you'll have to decide who gets to go first. Still, when it's his turn to come you'll enjoy feeling him bury his face in your pussy as it happens, even though you probably won't come along with him. It will be your turn next time.

All the Trimmings

If you perform a good blow job in the way we discussed above and put all your heart into it, you will already be better at it than 90% of women. If there was any justice in this cold, hard world of ours, you would be entitled to some form of recognition. You should be at least a Black Belt (1st Dan) in Fellatio and should have less talented women stopping you in the street to ask for advice. As it is, only your man will really be able to sing your praises, and I bet you would prefer him to keep quiet. (Strange, isn't it? You like him to say things like 'My wife's a fantastic cook' or 'Her 400m meter hurdles record is within a second of the Olympic qualifying time'. At your next dinner party, why can't he say 'Her playing of the pink oboe is so magical she deserves a Congressional Medal of Honor'?)

Enough of that. What you want to know is, how do you add to your skill and finally reach that coveted 7th Dan for your Black Belt?

Perhaps the most important thing – and the most difficult to master – is the reading of his excitement so you can respond with just the right speed and intensity to make him do what you want. It is this instant feedback that piles layer upon layer of sensation on your man. You get most of your information by listening to his breathing and sighing. The tensing of muscles and the swelling of his cock will also help you know what is happening. Reading the signs can be a difficult problem with a new lover, but the answer is the same – you need lots and lots of thoughtful practice. Your lucky man! Not only will he get lots of blow jobs, but at the end of it all he will have a world-class fellatrix sleeping next to him.

Some small tips:

- with him as far into your mouth as you can manage, try humming in your throat. A subtle vibration will come through to him and that's fun.

- again with him far into you, relax your mouth and move your head in a figure-of-eight motion as you slide him slowly out and back in again. Very pleasant.

- look him in the eyes as you do nice things to his cock. Unlike some women who feel too embarrassed to watch him munching on their pussy, your man likes to see your sexy eyes as you suck his cock.

- keep a spicy cough pastille in your mouth as you suck him. The best sort – were they designed for the job? – are Fishermen's Friends. Made in England for fishermen sailing into the stormy North Atlantic, these fiery lozenges will make him feel as if he is stirring a chilli con carne with his cock.

- if you are feeling excited, make excited noises. When you take it out for a rest say things like 'I love sucking your cock' or 'I'm going to suck your balls dry, lover'. He wants to know that you are getting hot as well.

Try stroking his perineum (the area between his balls and his anus) while you suck him. He'll enjoy that, and if he seems open to it, you can go a little further. His anus has lots of nerve endings and brushing him in that area is very stimulating. (It is also very naughty, and that definitely adds to the fun.) Try drenching your finger with baby oil and pressing against his back door. You can do this with the same rhythm as your stroking and licking, or much faster if you like.

And then there is the postilion (or postillionage). My dictionary says a postilion is 'a rider on a near-side horse drawing a coach etc. when there is no coach-driver'. I don't know how that relates to lovemaking but the name also means the practice of sticking your finger into his anus while you play with his cock. If he has reacted positively to your provocation, take a big dip of personal lubricant (better than baby oil) on your fingertip and rub it over and into his anus. He will love feeling your finger push inside, and you may not have time to do much else before he comes. After you have got a little way in, pull out and take some more lubricant. Then try again and push in as far as you can, at least past the second knuckle. This will be the only time he has felt 'full' in the sense that you feel full with a cock inside you, and he'll enjoy the sensation. Assuming you have put your finger in with the palm of your hand facing his balls, move your finger in a beckoning motion. By doing this you are massaging his prostate gland and this is very, very pleasurable. With practice he can come by this alone.

Deep Throat

And finally – Deep Throat. This is the trick of accepting his cock completely into your mouth. Given that an average cock is 5 or 6 inches long (12-15 cm) and your mouth is only 3 to 4 inches deep (8–10 cm), it is clear that you just cannot fit a normal cock into a normal mouth.

What you can do, with a little practice, is half swallow him so that his cock reaches into your throat. Why would you want to do this? It's not because you think he will enjoy it (although it is a nice extra) but because you like his cock so much that you want to swallow it right up. Take every last bit of his cock into your mouth and bury your nose in his pubic hair. Even lick his balls at the same time. Wow!

How difficult is it? I think of it as like learning how to ride a bicycle; a bit of a struggle at first but then suddenly it's easy. You need to learn the old sword-swallower's trick of relaxing your throat to let his cock in. And the best way to learn? You guessed – practice.

Practicing on his cock is not bad, but you will probably feel more comfortable starting by yourself with a suitable dildo. Sit down, get comfortable and try to swallow as much as you can of the dildo. As you reach the back of your mouth, you will immediately feel uncomfortable. When this happens, pull the dildo back a fraction, swallow and try again. You will find getting to the beginning of your throat is not too difficult; just keep swallowing and trying to relax and you will be surprised how far you can get.

As you are sitting in your armchair and probing with the dildo, you are putting it in more or less horizontally – the natural angle of your mouth. However your throat runs down your neck and is vertical, and you will have the most success if you tip your head back so mouth and throat are in line. Take things easy and keep trying to swallow the dildo into the beginning of your throat. You might gag or cough, but just pull it back, swallow to relax, and keep trying. If you try to stick your tongue out at the same time, you will widen the back of your mouth and help progress. It feels a bit stupid doing this by yourself, and it will probably make your eyes water, but in the end it is worth the effort.

With a little practice you'll find yourself swallowing the tip of the dildo past the constriction that marks the beginning of your throat. There! You've done the difficult bit. Keep experimenting and you'll find you can finally get the head of the dildo into your throat, and leave it there until you need to breathe. You should be able to get this far with a week or so of practice. But keep trying; your aim now should be to get comfortable with a cock deep inside for longer and longer periods.

The first time you try this with your man, you'd better warn him in advance. You need his co-operation because the last thing you need when you're swallowing him is any pushing on his part. I can guarantee his enthusiastic support for your efforts, because he knows the results will be very interesting to him. Make sure you have control of what is happening. Try laying him on his side and approaching him across the bed. That way you can move around and line up your throat easily.

You will find swallowing a real cock is easier than a dildo, because the head is softer and more yielding. The enjoyment you get from taking him all into your mouth will be increased by the impression you will make on him. We all thrive on a little genuine admiration now and then. Mix deep throating in with your normal technique. If you time it right and are confident of his self-control, you can swallow him as he comes; there will be no question of swallowing his come or not – it will be heading straight south and you won't even taste it.

Once you are truly proficient, you will be able to do it from any angle and you will have the pleasure of swooping down on his cock and gliding down to bury your nose in his hair all in one movement. You will certainly be a big league fellatrix then!

Let me stress again that it's not necessary to master deep throat technique in order to give memorable oral sex. There are so many other sucks, kisses and caresses you can give that missing this one from your bag of tricks is not disastrous. And just to keep things in proportion, deep throating is not about him working his cock in your mouth and throat until he comes. You do not want your skilful mouth used as a substitute vagina. You swallow him because you enjoy having all that lovely cock in your mouth. And he will enjoy it too.

- 10 -

If a thing is worth doing, it is worth doing
slowly . . . very slowly.
Gypsy Rose Lee

A woman who has the divine gift of lechery and loves her partner will
masturbate him well – subtly, unhurriedly and mercilessly.
Dr Alex Comfort

The Search for the Perfect Hand Job

It's a fair bet that the first time you got your man really excited, you did it by hand – even if you finished him off some other way. It's the natural way for you to stimulate him; just make a grab for his cock. After all, he's been doing the same since he was twelve and it works for him. In previous generations many couples did no more than this before marriage. A secret hand job in the back seat of the car or the back row of the cinema was the most they could hope for.

With so many other things for a modern couple to do, the old-fashioned hand job has lost some of its charm. It is not seen as a sexual technique in its own right, and is thought of as very much a second-class experience. In the professional world it is seen differently. Workers in massage parlours (read 'stress relief centres' in my town) have traditionally offered a hand job as an extra, either legally or illegally. The reason for this is that hopping up onto the massage table to sit on your client's spike could be very compromising (and almost certainly illegal). And oral sex is much less attractive to the masseuse because it is too intimate and takes too long. As a result, proficient masseuses have learnt to make their hand jobs as satisfying as possible. That way they get better tips, and their customers will ask for them again on their next visit.

Of course, you can do it much better than the professionals. You don't have any pressure of time, you are intimately acquainted with the cock you're working on and – above all – you love your man and are doing it with your heart as well as your hands.

Getting Started

You probably don't appreciate just how nice your hands feel to a man. They are smaller than his, more delicate and usually softer. The sensation of your hands holding and fondling his equipment is something he cannot give himself. You might be surprised that he prefers your fumbling and uncertain hands to his own, but that's what the magic is all about. With your hands he never knows exactly what is coming next and the anticipation is thrilling.

Generally, start by reaching for his cock. There may be times when you both enjoy teasing and stroking as you work your way closer and closer to his cock, but for the most part he will appreciate feeling you holding him right from the beginning. It might be hard or soft, or somewhere in between, but as you hold and fondle it you will feel his erection growing until it is the rigid pole that you know and love. Now you are free to explore the area. He wants to feel your hands everywhere, up and down his shaft, through his hair, cupping his balls and sliding deep between his legs. Don't neglect his cock while you do this, he wants it all.

He knows how he feels as you do this, but he doesn't have any idea of what is going through your mind. So talk to him. Not about the kids' Little League practice or the price of carrots, but about his cock and how much you are enjoying playing with it. Tell him how it looks to you as squeeze and tease, and pull his foreskin back if he still has one. Now is a good time to slip in a few compliments on its length and thickness, and to tell him how delightful it feels when you sit on it and it fills your pussy right up. Experiment a little with what levels of stimulation he can tolerate and what he really enjoys. He will find it easier to answer your questions when he is not too excited.

After you have got him hard and aroused, it's time to settle down to the business in hand. Lay him flat on his back and sit on his chest, with your back to him. His arms could be down by his sides, but he might be tempted to interfere with your work so it is better if he puts his hands behind his head. That way he is limited to stroking your back or reaching round to cup your breasts; his cock and your busy hands are out of reach. Sit well up on his chest with your tail close to

84

his chin; you won't hurt him and you will give your hands and arms more freedom of movement.

Tying him Down

You can give your man a very good time by sitting on his chest and slowly masturbating him. However, he is a strong and powerful animal and far from controllable by little old you. If he gets too excited you may just be tipped out of your comfortable saddle as he threshes around. Far better to tie him down; then he will be at your mercy and you can torment him at your leisure.

The easiest way to do this is to lay him on his back with his knees up. Spread his knees wide and cross his ankles. Now take one of his belts and tie his ankles together. You will need to wind the belt round at least twice before you can fasten it. It doesn't need to be very tight; firm is good enough. This is quite a clever tie-down because, as his ankles are crossed, he can neither close his knees nor straighten his legs. With his legs out of action you stand some chance of holding him down by your weight on his chest. It is also easy to achieve – you don't have to run down to your local sex shop to buy special equipment.

The alternative is to buy some proper restraints. Forget ropes and handcuffs; those are old-fashioned and need some skill to use quickly and effectively. The modern approach is to use wide straps secured on the wrists and ankles by Velcro. The straps incorporate metal rings that can be tied to the corners of your bed (or anywhere else you chose to torment him). Don't feel shy about buying them; they are very common and widely used. Your man will feel very excited when you poke him in the ribs at the sex shop and whisper that you want him to buy some. He might be imagining that he is going to use them on you but hey – what's sauce for the goose, is sauce for the gander!

All Yours

Regardless of whether or not you want to restrain him, when you sit on his chest there will be no doubt in his mind about who is in charge. His cock is right in front of you, ready for you to do whatever you want. The first thing to do is to make sure you have some baby oil or slippery hand cream nearby. It is better to use an oil-based product for this job as the water-based ones tend to dry out if exposed to the air for too long. (One of the main attractions of the water-based personal lubricants is that they are condom friendly. For your current operation you don't need a condom so a good slippery oil is just fine. Just dollop it on as required.)

Start gently by touching and caressing his cock and balls until he is rigid and then vary your techniques a little to give him a range of different pleasures. With a thumb and forefinger squeezing a ring around the base of his cock, pull down until your hand is in his hair and the skin is tight. You can use the other fingers of this hand to cup his balls (carefully). Now the head of his cock is stretched, shiny and very hungry, and you are ready to start. Take some oil on the fingers of your other hand and try the following:

-    form your thumb and forefinger into a ring that fits tightly over the widest part of the glans. Move it slowly up and down, forcing his glans through the ring on each stroke coming and going. This works wonders with the sensitive rim and the shaft just below.

-    make a sort of mouth with all of your fingers and thumb and push it over his glans. Vary the direction you approach him in, and pretend it is some sort of animal swallowing him up.

-    still with the skin held firmly back, grasp the base of the shaft tightly with your other hand and slide it back up the shaft. Repeat this, moving all the time in the same direction. When you've done that for a while, reverse the direction.

-    force your fist over the head and down to the shaft. As this fist is now pulling down on the shaft, release your other hand and use it to follow the first, and so on. As your fists slide over him one after the other, he will feel as if he is continuously penetrating the tightest of vaginas.

-    check to see if you can unscrew the head of his cock. When he is quivering in exquisite agony, say 'Well, maybe it's a left-hand thread.' and try in the opposite direction.

-    roll the shaft vigorously between your two palms, like a boy-scout trying to start a fire.

-     with one finger, swirl round and round the glans, making sure to catch the rim in particular.

If you can think of any other interesting caresses to use, now is the time to try them.

The Main Course

This is where you settle down to the main course. Your object here is to give continuous rhythmic stimulation, working towards an orgasm but denying him relief at the last minute.

Give him about twenty quick strokes, each spaced at intervals of about a second. That is, the individual strokes are fast but you space them out slowly. Then give him a rapid burst of ten continuous fast strokes. Follow with another twenty strokes at one second intervals and so on. Treating him like this will start him inevitably on the golden road to orgasm, but before he gets there, stop and let him cool down before resuming your torture. Not many men can stand much of this and within ten minutes he will be begging you to let him come. If you can stretch it out to fifteen minutes without an accidental orgasm, it means that not only are you becoming very clever, but you also enjoy torturing helpless animals.

Ejaculation

Every girl enjoys watching her man come. It's very exciting to see that he is completely out of control, and that all his heart, personality and intelligence are concentrated for that instant in his cock and balls. It is even more fun if you know that this explosion has been brought about by little old you, using all the arts and skills of a courtesan of legend.

When the Great Moment arrives, all the machinery starts working at once, all in irreversible, automatic mode. You will feel all his muscles tense and his cock seems to become harder and even bigger. The glans is swollen to its limit and its colour is more intense. Then deep in the roots of his cock and balls a series of violent contractions start. They are remarkably consistent from man to man in coming at 0.8 second intervals. (Even clearer proof that some-one up there loves us is that your own contractions during orgasm come at exactly the same frequency – orgasms don't come more simultaneous than that.) The contractions force the sperm and carrying liquid up the big 'vein' running up the lower side of his cock and the mixture squirts into you – or up into the air in the case of your current hand job. You can feel all this happening more easily if you have your fingers around and behind his balls.

The amount of ejaculate varies. A normally hungry man having an orgasm after little foreplay will produce one or two teaspoons of thick white liquid. If you are giving him a second orgasm or you have made love not long ago, the amount will be reduced and might appear a little thinner because there is less sperm available in the carrying liquid. On the other hand, if your man has not made love for a couple of days, and you have invested time and skill in bringing him to the verge of orgasm several times before allowing him to come, he will produce more. The increase achieved this way will be mostly liquid rather than sperm, but who's counting? It is fun to watch it fountain out of him and more is better. And now you know how to maximize production.

Sometimes his come will be expelled with some force and can even carry a few feet, particularly with the first contraction. If you want to experiment with this, you need to have no restrictions to the flow of come at that instant. So keep your fingers away from the lower side of his cock – you don't want to press on the tube there – and point his cock at a natural angle away from his body so there are no kinks to restrict the flow. Not every man can do this so don't be disappointed if you don't have to clean the ceiling next morning.

If you are deliberately pressing on the tube, he will 'backfire'. This happens when the sperm, being denied an outlet in the normal way, is squeezed back up into the bladder. (In your misspent youth you may have noticed this if you ever made love to your boy friend while walking home, standing up against a wall or in the church porch – you know what I am talking about. If you pulled the waistband of your panty hose down and let him slide in between your lips from the front, you were probably surprised at how little mess there was to clean up when you got home. The waistband of your panty hose had been stopping the flow getting out.) While this seems to do no harm to him, it's not comfortable and it certainly detracts from the fun of watching the come spurting out over your hands, his tummy, the sheets, everywhere!

To intensify the feeling of orgasm, hold his glans tightly. Take just the glans in your fist, with the thumb side towards his body. With the rim of his glans circled by your thumb and forefinger and the rest of the glans reaching into the palm of your hand, squeeze hard in rapid pulses – try for the magic 0.8 of a second rhythm. You will need to be alert to what is happening if you are to start this at the right moment. Your first squeeze should start just as his first contraction hits and you should continue pulsing your fist at the same rhythm until nothing else is coming out. This is the same exercise I suggested for oral sex, when you cover your teeth and 'bite' the glans rapidly as he comes. And as I told you before, watch out for violent spasms through his whole body when you do this correctly.

What to do with the Mess?

It's not mess! It's his come, so don't scream and lunge for a tissue. Old wives say that come is good for the skin. I don't know whether I should believe them or not, but I think I will. So rub it on to your tummy and breasts, and tell him how nice it is. There's not much of it and it will dry quickly without leaving you sticky, although you will smell nicely of sex.

He will probably be floating with the birds after the tumultuous orgasm you have just given him, and it is unfair to expect much from him for a while. Sorry, but you were in charge and you should have arranged some satisfaction for yourself before starting such a magnificent hand job. Now you can only cuddle up to him and relax.

It is a nice and comforting thing for you to hold his cock and balls at times like these. He always enjoys feeling your delicate hand there. It adds to the experience and, you never know, you might find it growing hard again in your hand. There is an etiquette for dealing with this sort of revived erection. I refer you to Sheherezade and her stories of the great Caliph Haroun al-Rashid in the Arabian Nights. Two of Haroun's many slave-girls were arguing in the great man's bed over just such an erection until one said 'on the authority of

Hisham ibn Orwah, who had it of his grandfather, the Prophet said "Whoso quickens the dead, the dead belongs to him and is his.'" Even so, she didn't get to use the erection; her colleague seized it by force and took it as her own. And today the tradition still remains, if you can get it to stand up, it's yours to do what you want with. Just keep the other slave-girls and concubines away from it.

- 11 -

I love the idea of there being two sexes, don't you?
James Thurber

The essence of life is the smile of round female bottoms.
Guy de Maupassant

Hotting up

Where did we leave you and your man before you went off to your classes on oral sex and hand jobs? You had been using your sexy body to tantalize him, giving him the kind of personal, up-close lap dance that no professional would ever give him. Now it's time to show some mercy and let him get closer to that hot little pussy he's dying to investigate.

Women often love to lay back and have their bodies worshipped by a thoughtful lover, to be dominated and used until they are in ecstasy. Well, guess what? So do men. Of course they can't absorb anything like the pleasure women can, and surfing cloud nine for minutes at a time is unfortunately impossible, but they do like to try sometimes. Who gets to be boss in lovemaking is something you negotiate with your partner over time. For most active couples, one partner will take control more often than the other but all healthy couples change around. You may find yourself changing during the course of a lovemaking session – you've had your fun with me, now I'm going to have mine with you. There is no harm in one of you saying 'Tonight I'm calling the shots, so all you have to do is relax and enjoy it'. Most men find it very easy to go along with a proposition like that.

After the long and luxurious teasing you have been giving him, your man wants your pussy, so I suggest you give it to him. Lay him on his back on the floor with his head near a chair arm or similar. Putting his arms by his sides, kneel over his chest again and shuffle slowly forward. As your pussy gets closer and closer he is going to be afraid that you will stop just out of licking range again, but this time you can be kind to him.

Once you are within reach, he will make a dive for your pussy. This is fine but you need to show him who is the boss so press down on his forehead to hold him away. Now with his head still on the floor, start brushing against his mouth with your pussy. He will probably offer his tongue immediately but even if he does say something like 'Oh, lick me lover – lick me!' and move carefully around so that all the places you like to get licked are brought to his tongue. It will be better for both of you if you can avoid coming immediately; there's plenty of time for that and he really does want to lick, kiss and suck every juicy bit of you.

Once he understands that he is not to move anything other than his tongue, you can rest your elbows on the chair arm in front of you and support your weight as you slide up and down, round and round. (While you are doing this, take a moment to reflect on my good advice about removing all the hair that is anywhere near your lips. His face and mouth would become sore very quickly if you were rubbing him with a hairy pussy.) Exactly what you ask him to do to you will depend entirely on what you enjoy most. As well as giving him the places you want stimulated, tell him what to do; lick, suck, poke – he won't know unless you tell him. Some women want rough treatment of their clit right from the start, others want it only at the last minute. He will be fascinated with the entrance to your vagina and if you like feeling his tongue inside you, tell him. Other women find this dull or even irritating. Before you get too carried away, look down at him and try to explain how wonderful he is making you feel. Don't cut your time on his face short; he is enjoying himself and you wouldn't want to deprive him, would you?

As you look at his face between your thighs, half obscured by the pussy you are pressing against his mouth, you might think he looks uncomfortable. Believe me he is not; he is actually in male heaven. He is immensely excited by what you are doing to him because everyone likes to be used for their lover's pleasure sometimes. You will feel he is breathing through the corners of his mouth as you partially smother him; it's a trick that lovers of pussy soon learn. The only way you can really hurt him down there is with your pubic bone, the ridge of bone crossing just above your pussy. If you were to press this on his nose and rest all your weight on it, you would find yourself instantly thrown across the room. This is slightly more of a problem if you are facing the other way and rest your weight on his chin. You could dislocate his jaw. That is why it's a good idea to have something in front of you to take your weight, like a chair arm. If there is nothing convenient, try the following. Put a small, very firm cushion under the top of his head (a bigger one doubled up will do) so that he is looking down over his chest. Now get on all fours over him with your head towards his feet and shuffle backwards until you can kiss his face with your pussy. The cushion will have lifted his head to the right angle and you can continue as before. This position is second best; you have less freedom of movement, you can't see his eyes, and he won't feel so dominated, but it's still good fun for both of you.

Back to being on top of him. You have been sliding around so that he is probably wet from ear to ear by now. It's time to take a little pleasure yourself, so concentrate on what brings you to orgasm. It might be as simple as just licking your clit, or you might want it sucked and licked at the same time. Try gently rubbing your clit on the end of his nose and enjoying his tongue inside you at the same time. Do whatever turns you on, and don't stop until it does.

When you have come, shuffle back down him and enjoy a kiss and a cuddle. A kiss? When he's all wet with me? Yuck! Yuck nothing. You should be ashamed of yourself. After all the nice things he's been doing for you and you don't even want to share a kiss with him? Oh well, just give his mouth a quick wipe with your hand, but kiss him anyway. He deserves it.

Women and the Silent Orgasm

Some women moan and shout in the throes of orgasm. Not very many, and far less than porno films would have you believe. In fact having a very noisy lady is inconvenient for a man. He probably doesn't mind who hears her, but she does. The fear of being overheard when out of control is so strong in many women that their lovemaking is limited to soundproof rooms or wilderness spaces.

On the other hand, no man wants a completely silent lover. This is not because he enjoys the noise (he does) but because unless he can hear what's happening to you, he doesn't know if you're enjoying it. Imagine: he licks your clit and nothing happens. What does he do next? Or on the other hand he licks your clit and is rewarded by a sharp intake of breath and a sigh. Now there is no doubt what to do next, and he is going to keep doing it with an enthusiasm matching the signals you are sending him. For your man the most rewarding thing about your orgasm is the feedback that makes him part of the process. For him there is nothing worse than working alone on a semi-comatose woman until she suddenly looks up and says 'Stop – I've come'.

If your man takes over the kitchen and makes you an apple pie, would you dream of saying thank you and take it off to eat all by yourself? Of course not; you would automatically share it with him. Well, the orgasms he makes for you are just the same; he deserves a share and you should ask yourself whether you are being selfish when you come.

Women come in many different ways and here I suggest you look at a website called www.cdgirls.com. This is an interesting site and differs from the normal run of adult material. Although they have branched out into other things recently, the site seems to have been based on two interesting ideas. Firstly the Sybian Rider, which is a fascinating and overwhelming invention. It looks a bit like a small, saddle-shaped stool with an artificial cock sticking up in the middle. The idea is that you sit on the saddle with your knees on the floor and the cock inside you. The operator switches it on and you find that not only does the cock vibrate, it also rotates in a stirring motion inside you. The speed of both vibration and rotation are variable and a skilled operator can take you in five minutes from a pleasantly sexy feeling to having so many continuous orgasms that you fall over.

Very interesting, but the special twist that CDGirls brought to their website – the second interesting idea – is that they used normal girls on their machine, and told them to relax and act naturally while they were filmed enjoying themselves. The results are 100% real and show just how variable women's orgasms can be. They have built up a considerable and rewarding archive of different orgasms. I suggest you (and your man) visit the site and take a month's subscription, all in the interest of science of course. Try looking at the video of Mimi, a pretty blonde. She sits on the Sybian and once she is comfortable, closes her eyes and starts coming. Eventually the machine is turned off and her eyes open again. Apparently she has just experienced a series of shattering orgasms, and the operator persuades her, after a short break, to hop back on the machine and do it again. This time she closes her eyes and reaches a climax much more quickly (we think). Again her eyes don't open again until the machine is switched off.

Watching Mimi has been very interesting, but now try Aspen, an elegant brunette with an outgoing personality. She installs herself on the Sybian and you can immediately see from her sighs and her movements that something good is beginning to happen. And happen it does. Without the extravagant noises and comment of the porno industry, it is quite clear that Aspen is having the ride of her life until she can't take any more and gets off.

Try other videos and you will be surprised at how different women can be. If you want to study in detail the interaction of the operator and the subject, try the video of Jade, an Asian girl who is one of CDGirls best operators. She installs herself on an interesting double dildo and there follows a remarkable sequence of stimulation and orgasm, created between experts, until she says she has had enough. Apparently, she has never said that before.

Apart from being very exciting for both you and your man to watch, the videos will give you some understanding of the difficulties he faces. If you are naturally very quiet and still as you come, he just won't know what is happening. And if he doesn't know what effect his caresses are having, he won't be able to refine them and direct them in precisely the best way for you.

So what can you do to help him play your body like a concert piano? Don't force yourself to act in any way other than naturally; that would be counterproductive. You can talk to him before you become incoherent, and you should make yourself do this. It's not difficult to say 'Ooh – that's good!' or 'Yes, that's just the right place. Harder!' In fact after you have forced your lady-like lips to say these things a couple of times, you will find yourself saying them without thinking. The most difficult time is when you are lying there incoherent from ecstasy. It is impossible to think, let alone speak. Try starting off by breathing through your mouth so he can hear you panting, and with luck you will continue panting even when you are out of control. If you feel at all like making a sound, encourage yourself to make it. Don't try and force things – you'll only spoil your orgasm for both of you – but if there is something you can manage easily, do it. You don't have to make a noise; movement is just as good. If you can set up a rhythmic movement of your hips while he is licking you, he will pick up signals from the way you move that will help him give you what you need, exactly as hard and as fast as you need it. You can also send signals through your hands. Hold his head and I am sure you will find yourself pulling him into your pussy as it all happens. If he is making you come by hand, rest your own hand on the back of his neck or his cheek; you will be surprised at what he can read through your fingertips.

Riding Him

By now, getting inside you will have become the most important thing in your man's mind, and your time for teasing him is drawing to an end. On the other hand, you know from experience that riding up and down on top of him is likely to result in a very quick end to your fun. Instead of putting him inside you straight away, try laying his cock on his stomach and sitting on the base of it and his balls.

This is called 'Riding the Broomstick' and puts witchcraft in a new light. In this position your pussy is kissing the shaft of his cock and your wet lips are surrounding him. He will be watching you enjoying yourself, and your excitement will add to his own. If you can manage it, play with your breasts. Of course that will feel nice, but can you imagine how hot it will look to him?

By leaning forward in this position you will be able to put as much weight as you like on your pussy, and you can directly stimulate your clit by moving backwards and forwards. He will enjoy your thrusting too, but the stimulation will be indirect and more bearable. If you want to increase the level of his stimulation, move up his cock so that you are rubbing his glans. He will love the luxurious feeling of your smooth, wet pussy pressing and sliding on his glans. (If you have been a bad girl and forgotten to clean the hair well away from your lips, this movement could be the last you make before he fills his navel with come.) Be careful not to be too rough with him, but by all means rub your clit against his shaft as much as you like. Come if you want to – why not? There are plenty more orgasms where that came from.

In the end, you want him inside you and now is the time. Sink onto him, and you will both be on automatic pilot. After all the loving attention you have been giving him for the last few hours, I can't imagine you will have a long ride.

- 12 -

Believe me, my young friend, there is nothing – absolutely nothing – half so much worth doing as simply messing about in women.
with apologies to Kenneth Grahame

'How about it, Sis – I mean, like can you come on top?'
'You silly-billy,' she chided, 'I can come on card tricks!'
Terry Southern Blue Movie

The Wonderful Female Orgasm

If you have been a good student, you carefully followed the suggestions in previous chapters on teasing, tantalizing and finally rewarding your man. You might be surprised that you have spent nearly all your time on the build up, and hardly any time at all on the last ascent to your man's orgasm. But I am sure you did not get any complaints, so you must have done the right thing. However, you don't want to do the same thing all the time, so keep the full treatment for special occasions and just use the ideas you have read about as you need them. You don't want to serve your man like a concubine every day; he might get lazy. For normal times you need more equitable arrangements.

You know that the overall goals of lovemaking are to have fun and express your love for each other (forget about the few occasions in your life when you do it to make babies), but have you thought about what you are aiming at during the act itself? You might be aiming at quick, mutual relief, as in having a quickie in a phone booth on the way home. However most lovemaking takes place in more controlled circumstances, so what are you trying to do then? Well one thing you should never do is start lovemaking to give only one of you an orgasm. Usually the man. Using your pussy to give him pleasure without taking any yourself is an act of charity – cold and condescending. Bad for you, bad for him and bad for your relationship. If he wants to come and you don't, then masturbate him or, better still, encourage him to do it himself. (It is important that you are part of this so don't turn your back and tell him to get on with it. You still love him even if you are not feeling horny tonight, so rest your head on his shoulder, cup his balls with your hand and feel him make himself come. You can even volunteer to take over for the last seconds. The important things are that he is happy, you have not been pushed into something you didn't want and you both did it together.)

In fact the main aim of lovemaking is to give the woman the orgasms she wants. And the secondary aim is to prepare her to enjoy her man's orgasm.

These two things are what successful lovemaking is all about, and the description covers all the different things you might want to do to each other. You might think this sounds one-sided and that your man's orgasm is almost sidelined. For once, your own physiology proves you wrong. Why would we have been blessed with the ability to have lots of long orgasms if we weren't meant to enjoy them? If women had been designed to have a single, sharp orgasm like a man, things would be different. Then the goal of lovemaking would be a single, simultaneous orgasm. As things are, you need and are entitled to a long build-up – with orgasms – before joining in your man's climax. Of course you can have some sympathy for men as they seem to be getting much less out of it than you are, but don't cry too hard. You didn't make the rules, and women have to put up with a lot of things that would make a man give up in disgust.

In fact, he enjoys giving you orgasms. Men find it very satisfying to watch and feel a woman break down and come, and the more orgasms you share with him, the more he enjoys it. Of course, you probably won't join him when he finally comes. You can't get it right all the time, but his orgasm is much more satisfying for you if you are still glowing from yours.

Being Orgasmic

Being orgasmic is very important for you, and you shouldn't be put off with anything less. If you are having trouble coming, don't worry, there is plenty of good news for you. Importantly, if you can come at all then you can be sure that there is nothing physically wrong with you, and your enjoyment of more orgasms is simply a matter of physical practice and mental attitude. But having only rare or occasional orgasms is a terrible thing because it will colour your relationship with your man. No relationship suffers from a good and active sex life but most can be diminished by a lack of good lovemaking.

The first thing to remember is that hardly anyone comes regularly through intercourse alone. Even the cleverest and sexiest women need some help. They are careful to have their orgasms early through foreplay and oral sex, and that makes it a bit easier to come with their partner's cock, but still there is no guarantee. So you're not alone.

Remember, I am not a doctor so I'm not going to offer medical advice but I can say that if you never come you really need to discuss things with your man and look for help. Do it together if you can, because things are easier if you are both working on the problem. Fortunately nearly everyone can improve their love life with the right help.

If your problem is just that you find it difficult to come, then things are much easier, especially if you have your man's help. Don't rush off for expensive counselling; the answer lies in your own hands. Firstly, can you come easily when you masturbate? If you can then you really have no significant difficulty at all. Just incorporate masturbation into your lovemaking and you have an instant fix to the problem. Of course you need your man's co-operation but that is not going to be difficult to get as long as he knows what you are trying to do. You just need to use a suitable position for lovemaking. The classic missionary position is not so good because your hand will be trapped between the two of you. Woman on top (cowgirl) is not bad because when sitting on him you have free access to your clit, and as a bonus you can look into each other's eyes. However he cannot do much to help you in this position because you are too close. Doggy position gives you and him very good access, but it can be a bit lonely unless you are doing it in front of a big mirror so you can see each other.

Perhaps the best is the Lazy Sunday Morning position. Lie on your back with your right knee raised. He lies at right angles to you, under that raised knee, and holds your left thigh squeezed between his. (Of course, you can switch the lefts and rights.) In this position he is well placed to slip into you, and both of you are so relaxed that you could fall asleep if you didn't have other things on your mind. Both of you have easy access to your clit and while he moves gently in and out, you can be working on it in turns or even together. As he gets more practice (and provided you are telling him how to do it), he will learn exactly what you need for your orgasm. Although you are probably better at the build up to orgasm, it is nice to have his help while you're actually coming because he isn't out of his mind with ecstasy and can draw things out much more satisfactorily. You can also use a vibrator in this position (see below) and that is a guaranteed way of coming if the atmosphere is right.

Changing your Mind

The other common problem is the woman who can generally come when she puts her mind to it, but takes a long time to get there. She struggles and struggles, but if there is the slightest distraction, Tonight's Show is Cancelled. This is probably more of a mental thing than a physical one. Stimulation by hand as above will probably help but that doesn't address fundamental problems because in the end all we are talking about there is stimulating your clit more efficiently. If your partner is rubbing and rubbing for half an hour while you frantically try to rearrange your thoughts into orgasm mode, you are probably talking about a deeper problem.

I read an article by a woman who just could not enjoy oral sex with her eyes open or the light on. She could not bear the sight of a man eating her pussy. The fact was that she disliked herself so much that she could not understand how anyone would want to put his face near her pussy, let alone kiss it. And then one day a lover was munching happily away on her when he looked her in the eye and winked. That just finished her; she could not come at all that day.

If you are one of the women who through upbringing or conviction suspect that sex is dirty and sinful, it can be difficult to relax with your own sexuality and enjoy what is happening. If you are really unhappy imagining your body as a sex object for your partner, it is hard to surrender yourself to him. If you are one of these unfortunate women, I bet you have read this far with interest but thinking that none of it applies to you. Well, you're wrong. I am not a raging pervert – well, not all the time anyway – and the ideas and attitudes I have been writing about are normal, mainstream, ice-cream-and-apple-pie common sense. In fact I will go further; if you have trouble relaxing during sex and you also can't see any of the book applying to you, you only have two choices if you want a long and contented future. Either join a nunnery and forget your problems, or start taking the idea of sexual attractiveness seriously. Don't ever say to yourself 'I try to come but it's too difficult so I don't bother'. Do something about it, and start today. You owe it to yourself, and you owe it to your man.

I am sure you have seen films where a few young men are taken off the streets, stood up in a courtyard and shouted at. They look a pretty sorry lot until they are sent off to the quartermaster to get their uniforms. When they get back they look better, they stand taller and they feel better about themselves. They have already started to be soldiers; just putting on the uniform has started to change the way they think. You need the same sort of transformation. Start dressing and behaving like an attractive woman, and pretty soon you'll be thinking like one. And then you'll realize that you are an attractive woman and your prize will be – after a little enjoyable practice – a satisfying love life complete with orgasms, even earthshaking ones if you study hard.

I suggest you make yourself a list of achievable targets for the coming month with the aim of changing the way you dress and present yourself. Again, I mean really make a list – don't just sit and read about it. Imagine yourself as the attractive and sexy woman you want to be and work towards it, ticking off each promise as you achieve it. It's difficult to make such a list by yourself, and perhaps you should enlist the help of a girl friend and do it together (separate lists of course – everyone is different). You will need to push yourself a little – there will be no sense of achievement if everything is easy and comfortable. Just changing the colour of your Sloppy Joe sweater is definitely achieving nothing; you need to throw it out and get something that fits. Oh, and by the way, you had better keep your man informed or he will think the changes are due to your taking a new lover. Start week one something like this :-

Monday

1. Make hairdresser's appointment for a style my man will like

2. Make long appointment with beauty salon to learn again about selection and application of make-up

Tuesday

1. Buy new bras and thongs that are more sexy than comfortable

2. Prepare boring clothes for charity shop

Wednesday

1. Buy a (very) short casual skirt for weekends etc.

2. Pump my man to find one sexy thing I can do for my appearance that I'm not doing now

And so on. Be more daring for the next week. If you don't have any real heels, buy some. Promise to do things you are uncomfortable with, like wearing a see-through blouse with no bra around the house all evening. I don't care if you like your breasts or not (he doesn't care either), it's a sexy thing to do so swallow your doubts and just do it. Of course it is permitted to ask him how he likes the treat you're giving him, and welcome any suggestions he might have.

By the end of the third week you should have reworked your wardrobe – not completely, of course, unless you are unusually rich – and be promising yourself to do things like wear short skirts out shopping and putting your hand in his pants while driving around town.

The fourth week should be really pushing your limits. Go out with him in a skirt as short as you dare and no panties or panty hose (stockings are permitted). Book yourself in for a Brazilian wax job. Cook his dinner wearing only a tee shirt and apron. At the end of the week demand a celebration dinner and promise to pay for it by dressing like an elegant tart and making love to him all night.

At the end of the month, sit down with your girlfriend and compare notes. Concentrate on how much you've changed your thinking during the past month. In particular think about any great successes you had doing naughty things, and about how much you enjoyed it. It's good to look back at how you used to be and how far you've come. Of course, it is your man who should give the ultimate stamp of approval; does he find you more attractive than a month ago? If you have been honest with yourself, there will be no question.

I hope you also like the change. You are still the same intelligent person that you were before. You haven't lost your brain and turned into a bimbo just because you are wearing blouses that invite men to look down your cleavage. The question is, are you and your man having more fun? I am sure that if you are having more fun in general, you will be starting to have more fun in bed too. It won't happen overnight, of course, but keep trying to look attractive and sexy, and things can only get better and better.

The thing to remember about solving the orgasm problem is that it lies in your attitudes about yourself as a sexual person, and that if you are not relaxed with yourself no amount of rubbing is going to achieve anything other than blisters. You still need to be turned on, and so does he, so follow the ideas in this book about building sexual attraction and tension. As you need his help, you can even let him read it as well. Once you get to bed, take the attitude that you are there to enjoy yourselves, not to scale Everest. If you don't manage a stream of orgasms at your first attempt, keep it for next time. Love, intelligence, communication and practice will get you there in the end - trust me!

It is very, very important that you realize that orgasms are not something that are created only in bed. You need to feel sexy and attractive and desired for a good love life, so start at the beginning and force yourself to do what is necessary to feel sexy and attractive. There are no alternatives, apart from giving up on your love life altogether. It really is up to you.

Toys

Toys are great fun - ask any kid - and adult toys are no different. A kid without toys is deprived, and if you have no toys in your bedroom drawer, what does that say about you? Are you so solemn that you never feel like playing? If you truly have no toys, sit on your man's lap tonight and get on the internet. Buying toys online is very easy although it is true that you have to wait for delivery. While you are waiting, hop in the car, get down to the nearest sex shop and buy something to be getting on with. Buying toys together is fun and you will especially enjoy the naughty feeling that everyone knows exactly what you are going to be doing as soon as you get home.

The classic toy, dating from the mists of time, is the dildo. This is an artificial cock made of whatever material is available. Nowadays ivory and wood are out of fashion and most of them are of a plastic gel. There are special ones that are exact marble replicas of some porn star's cock or are made of twirled Venetian glass, but most are of soft plastic. They come in a range of sizes, including very slim ones for use on your anus and ultra large ones that seem to be more imaginative than practical. Their major use is for your man to slide them in and out of you during oral sex. Having a cock inside you while your clit is being licked is very pleasant.

Nowadays, plain old dildos are pretty much out of favour and vibrators have taken over. The simplest vibrator is also an artificial cock, but it is a cock that gives you a vibratory massage as it slides over and into your pussy. It is very hard not to come with one of these throbbing on your clit, and a reliable vibrator has become standard equipment for many single women. They are also very popular with lovers; a man can do a lot more to you if he is armed with one of these magic toys.

A standard vibrator holds its batteries inside, rather like a flashlight. You switch it on and off, and vary the speed, by rotating the base. This can be a little difficult to do in the heat of the moment when your hands are slippery with baby oil, so you are probably better off with a vibe that has a separate control unit connected by a thin cable.

You will find there are very many different vibes, including ones that have a rotating motion as well as vibrating. The pearl and rabbit configuration is very popular; this type has a central section of rubbery plastic filled with beads, and a 'rabbit' figure with long ears projecting at an angle from the side, usually with its own small vibrator. The idea is that the pearls section sits just inside your entrance where the jiggling of the pearls feels good, and the rabbit is pressed between your lips, tickling your clit with his ears. Great fun. When choosing a cock shaped vibe, it is a good idea to go for one with a wide base. This makes it easier to set on a chair so you can sit on it. Then give your man the controls and let him buzz you to heaven while you try to lick him to orgasm before you become helpless.

Another class of vibe is the butterfly. These use a harness of panty elastic to hold a small vibrator against your clit. They can be worn during normal sex so you can have all the sensations at once. Yet another type is the egg, which is pretty much what it sounds like. You can use this as you fancy but one nice thing to do is to pop it deep inside you and let it vibe the end of your man's cock when he slides into you. You can even buy a radio-controlled egg; you hide it away inside you and your man carries the remote control in his pocket. Watch the faces of the other women in the supermarket checkout line or waiting at the bank. One of them might be struggling to conceal the nice things their lover is doing to them. Lucky lady!

The truth is, when it comes to vibrators you are overwhelmed by choice. What a delightful thought – it's going to take you years to work your way through all the different options.

Toys for Him

Are you surprised that nearly all the toys are for use on women? That reflects real life and the way good loving progresses. Toys are used to enhance foreplay and give the woman lots of orgasms before the man has his. If you brought home a toy that made your man come more quickly and effectively, what would you do for the rest of the evening? Play Monopoly? That is why the few male toys on sale are a focused on improving life for the single man rather than for use by a loving couple.

So if you want to buy your man an exciting toy, buy one that he can use to make you climb the walls.

Extras

And then there are all the other toys. Knobbly sheaths that slip onto his cock and torment your pussy with soft rubbery fingers. Straps that you tighten around his balls and the base of his cock that not only look exotic but also help maintain his erection. Pairs of hollow balls with loose weights inside them that that lie inside you and 'clunk' very satisfactorily each time you move. Ornaments that clip over your clit and allow you to show off your pussy complete with jewellery. And all sorts of massage oils and creams – the springs of human invention never run dry when there is something as absorbing as sex to think about. Try some, or try them all – I can guarantee you'll enjoy test-driving them.

- 13 -

It is impossible to obtain a conviction for sodomy from an English jury. Half of them don't believe that it can physically be done, and the other half are doing it.
Winston Churchill

Let's fool around. Let's do it some strange way that you've always wanted to, but nobody would do with you.
Manhattan the movie

Why Don't I just Slip into your Fantasy?

It is a well-established medical fact that the largest and most sensitive erogenous zone of your body is … your brain. The most important sexual stimulation is stimulation of the mind, and that is what we have been talking about for most of this book. You can achieve miracles by massaging his mind as well as massaging his cock. Offering your man a generous serving of pussy garnished with an imaginative dressing of fantasy is a sure way to his heart.

What is sexual fantasy? That's a huge question but I guess a simple answer is to say that fantasy covers all the exciting things that circulate in your imagination that you are not doing now. It can cover anything from beds of rose petals to being probed and examined by space aliens. The most intriguing feature of fantasy is that it might – just possibly – come true. That is what gives fantasy its spice.

Of course, fantasizing about aliens or film stars is further from reality than the sixteen year old boy imagining the chance to reach up the skirt of his sexy auntie, but they are all less likely to happen than winning the lottery. Still, the possibility is always there, and that is the essence of a good fantasy.

In an effort to give your man better lovemaking, you will soon find that there are limits to how much you can achieve merely by improving your technique. On the other hand, fantasy is unlimited.

So What can I Dream for You?

Most of your man's fantasies, and probably most of yours, are not so far out. Perhaps he dreams of seeing you in stockings and high heels, or taking you for dinner without your panties. These are things that you can easily give him and you will probably enjoy yourself as well. Then there are more daring things, like posing for nude photographs in public places, threesomes or anal sex. These you could manage but they might stretch your idea of where the line between normality and perversion lies. And then there are fantasies that you would never tolerate in a million years or ones that are just not physically possible, and I won't even start to think what they might be. You may be surprised that even this third category can be useful in sophisticated lovemaking.

The first thing to do with fantasies is to draw them out of your man's imagination. You can't do anything about them until you find out what they are. Handle this cleverly, and try and get the information out of him without letting on what you are doing. For instance, if you suspect that he has a yen to be tied up and tormented by a masked woman dressed in stockings and high-heeled boots, try casually surfing the internet with him and locate images like this. You know him well enough to tell from his reaction to photographs if there is something there that interests him.

The next step is to bring the idea up while you are making love. Take a break between orgasms and – preferably with him inside you – lead the conversation in that direction. Ask him why people like to be tied up during sex or what is it about stockings and boots that interest men. If you are a real artist you might get a lot of information out of him. Now you are ready to start building the fantasy situation, buying the boots, restraints and blindfolds you need.

Finally pick a day, give him a general warning that something good is coming and then surprise him. If you've planned well and are acting with your heart as you tie him down and tickle him with feathers (or whatever is on the menu at Madame Tutti's House of Fantasy), he will have a good time. More importantly, he will have something special to look back on. He will also be deeply in your debt and ready to repay you with a fantasy of your own.

Fantasies at this level are not for everyday use. Being blindfolded, covered in whipped cream and licked clean, is fine once in a while but it is fattening if indulged in too often. Most people's first reaction to having a fantasy fulfilled is – 'That was interesting' or 'That was fun'. You both go on to refine the fantasy, learn to do it better or longer until it becomes really pleasurable, and you then file it away for occasional revisits when the mood takes you.

Of course, by then your fertile brains will already be working out new fantasies; isn't the human mind a wonderful thing?

Sophistication or Perversion?

In your mind, some things are labelled as perversions. Where you draw the line is a personal thing and it is difficult to define. One definition of perversion is 'Something that gives the judge an erection'. My favourite definition from the book Foreign Affairs (written by a great thinker about sex – me) is 'Perversions are things that it would embarrass you to admit enjoying'.

Many States have legislated to outlaw 'perversions' and the results have been laughable. In theory if you are travelling around the US you had better call the local DA before indulging in oral sex (imagine how embarrassing a phone call like that would be!) because it is sometimes illegal. Gays and lesbians also ride the edge of legality. Some things are universally accepted as being beyond the boundary – child sex certainly, and striking up too close a relationship with your German Shepherd. (Although, interestingly, because you are female you might just slip the last one through in some jurisdictions. They couldn't even catch you for cruelty to animals, not after giving him the time of his doggy life.)

The changes in attitude brought by time are also interesting. In the US, England and the British Empire at the beginning of the twentieth century, a vigorous argument was raging over whether it was perverse for a widower to marry his dead wife's sister. Biblical references were trotted out and learned professors foamed at the mouth over … over what, for goodness sake? Who cares anymore? Attitudes to gays have also changed markedly, not because there has been change in right and wrong, but because society has begun to feel that it doesn't really matter. What people do with their private parts is no-one's business but their own. If you and your man are happy when he wanders around the house dressed in no more than a neatly tied bow of blue ribbon, go right ahead. That's what the Constitution is for.

What do such extreme things have to do with you? Well, just because you won't or can't make love in a horse-drawn carriage riding around Central Park, doesn't mean you can't dream about it. If you can peep into your man's fantasy world, you can talk about it to him as you make love, and encourage him to imagine what it might feel like to actually do some of these things. Talk about the sound of the horse's hooves, the cold wind on his naked butt, the swaying of the carriage. If you do it well he'll almost believe in it, and you will find the results are very gratifying.

Let your own reserve slip a little and trying sharing outrageous things from your own compendium of fantasies. He'll find it exciting to massage your imagination too.

And then there the attainable fantasies, the ones that are just a little beyond the range of your current activities and perhaps it is here that you will find your best opportunities for fun. Don't be afraid to experiment with any of the things below. They are done so widely that many people would define them as mainstream anyway. Having been tied up and tickled doesn't immediately transform you into a 'pervert'. The only thing you'll find out is whether or not it's as interesting as you had imagined. If it wasn't, don't do it again. If it was, well, lucky girl! So here are some common things you might like to try.

Bondage and SM Play

Bondage refers to tying someone up for sexual purposes. SM is short for Sado-Masochism, the giving and receiving of pain, again for sexual reasons. Note that we are talking about play here, NOT about the real thing.

If he is intrigued by the idea of tying you up, try buying a specialist magazine or surfing the net. Looking at pictures together will give you an idea of what your man is thinking and also give you a chance to tell him what you might be persuaded to try (and equally

111

important, what you definitely will not try). Once you have a picture of what's needed, you can start arranging the situation. But before you put the straps into his hands, work out some rules. Agree that nothing will ever be tied around the neck, and that no one will be left alone while tied up. Share a 'safe word' – a word like 'wheelbarrow' which if used means that the play-acting stops immediately and all bonds are untied. A safe word allows you to shout and scream and have your protests ignored by your villainous torturer – until you say the word and the villain turns back into a pussy cat.

Bondage can involve anything from tying your wrists to the bed head to trussing you up like a smoked ham. The complicated rope work is definitely for the experts, and you might come to that at some time in the future. (It's very difficult to do neatly and correctly, and takes so long you might fall asleep.) To start off, limit yourselves to the purpose-made ankle and wrist straps available in sex-shops. You will probably need some short lengths of rope or ribbons to tie the straps onto the corners of the bed. Once you've allowed him to spread-eagle you on the bed so that you can do no more than struggle against your restraints, he will probably want to blindfold you as well. Now he will start to 'torture' you, which usually means making you orgasm by tickling with feathers, by stroking with a shaving brush, by using a cucumber or a vibrator, licking you to death, whatever. As you are unable to stop him, you will no doubt find yourself 'forced' to come a surprising number of times.

You may want to be gagged. Gagging is a strange idea if you think about it, but the fact is that someone who is normally quiet and restrained can find themselves shouting and moaning into a gag – because no one can hear them. The sense of release the victim feels is remarkable. Of course, you need to agree something like finger clicking as a 'safe word' meaning that the gag should be removed. Ball gags are easily bought and effective. Do not try and make your own gag from panties or stockings; they might get accidentally sucked into the victim's mouth and make breathing difficult.

Note that I have been talking about being tied up and forced to enjoy having nice things done to you; the other side of the menu card includes restraining and discipline. We are not talking about flogging here; that is strictly for the extreme comic books. Nor are we talking about using whips, nipple clamps or any of the other painful instruments you can see in photographs – leave those for the experts. Much more common is spanking, usually on the butt. Don't reject this out of hand, because many women are surprised by a positive reaction when naughty things are done to their bottoms. The idea here is to be put over his knee and spanked with many blows that are harder than a pat but a little softer that the slap your mother used to give you when you were behaving badly. Continuous spanking spread all over your bottom will bring a glow to your cheeks and you may find yourself getting very wet indeed. Traditionally, your man will find an excuse to spank you – if you've been a bad girl – and will warm your bottom until he is convinced that you are truly sorry. He will then forgive you by making love to you, usually from behind where he can admire your pink cheeks.

Exhibitionism

Sum up exhibitionism as doing naughty things in public places. This is one activity that seems to be on the increase and for that you can blame the digital camera and the internet. The idea is that you both take off to a public place – say a park. He's brought a camera and you are dressed in shoes, a coat and nothing else. You take up a pose with a crowded footpath or a prominent landmark behind you and he takes your portrait – with your coat held invitingly open, of course. This is great fun, as you can imagine, and it is even more fun when you get home and swap pictures with other like-minded lunatics on the net. A variation is to go with a friend as well, and then your man can join you in even naughtier poses – I'll leave that to your imagination. Looking over your photo album with your man afterwards is an important part of the whole experience.

If you find exhibitionism exciting, let your man bribe or blackmail you into wearing very transparent clothing in public, maybe at a bar or a disco. Wear a transparent dress over fancy underwear and let the other men admire you. Finish your evening by going to the restroom and taking off the underwear. Walk back across the room mostly naked, pick up your coat and your man and leave. Can you imagine how excited you'll be feeling as you get to your car? They'll be talking about you in that bar for years, so you'd better pick one on the other side of town

Exhibitionism is legal everywhere – as long as no one sees you. In most of the US sharing your beautiful body with passers-by is definitely illegal, which is fair enough I suppose. No one should be forced into anything sexual, and if Mrs Normal wants to stay sexually dormant, that is her right. Exhibitionism seems more popular in Europe. You could always take a holiday in Holland or Germany where pictures of nude girls walking through shopping centres are becoming commonplace.

Piercing and Tattoos

Some people find piercing and tattooing exciting, not just the appearance but the whole process. Having designs tattooed on your skin, or rings and other metal objects stuck through unlikely places is a matter of taste. If you happen to like it, feel free. As a word of cold caution, never do it just because your partner will like it. This particularly applies to tattoos, which are by definition permanent. Of course, permanence is part of the whole mystique and enthusiasts consider semi-permanent transfers no substitute. I am by upbringing conservative in this area, but different people have different concepts of what is elegant, so it's their call. I like the idea of transfers because you can be decorative for a while, and then change your mind. I am attracted to small, intimate tattoos – the little man-in-the-moon at the top of your thigh, the discrete rose on the side of your butt, but perhaps I'm just an old fogey.

I also have trouble with rings in noses, but that is common with people who were brought up in the countryside a few years ago – the only ringed noses there belonged to pigs. If you are turned on by the sight of yourself in the mirror with unusual metalwork in your face, go ahead. We are talking about ornamentation that differs from having pierced ears only in degree, so perhaps I should appreciate it more. You can also pierce your nipples – quite common nowadays, and put rings through the inner lips of your pussy. Apparently these make no difference to sexual feelings but certainly look exotic.

There is just one piercing that does have sexual effects, and here I confess an unfulfilled interest. If you examine the hood of your clit and find that you can clean under it with a cotton bud, you have enough space for a vertical clitoral hood piercing. The object here is to insert a ring under the hood and out through a small piercing about a quarter inch (6 mm) up on the front. The ring sits vertically, and out of sight it is resting directly against your clit. Perhaps more popular than the ring is a small dumbbell – a bar with a ball on each end. The lower ball sits in the opening of your hood, and the top one embellishes the front.

A clitoral hood piercing looks pretty enough, and having the ring or dumbbell in direct contact with your clit adds a whole new level of stimulation during lovemaking. Apparently just walking around can be an interesting experience for the first few days. I wonder if I could get one as a birthday present?

Swinging, Threesomes and More

99.8% of men have dreamt about making love to two women at once. (You'll find the other 0.2% on the main streets and in the parks of our cities. They are called statues.) Many women dream of sex with two men but the figures are less certain here. Women tend to be – how shall I say it politely – economical with the truth when asked about this but I think it is clear that where the idea has occurred to them, it has occurred *with approval*. Two cocks at once would excite a saint.

This is certainly a very hot subject to talk about while making love. You can easily drive your man crazy by sitting on his cock and as you ride, explain to him how you would love to see a beautiful girl riding his tongue at the same time. Even if you hate the idea of touching another woman, you can always pretend for the duration of the fantasy. (I can't understand why you wouldn't want to experience another woman at least once. I can guarantee you will find it educational at the very least.) Ask him to explain how to make another woman come (as if you don't know!) or how you should play with her breasts. Piquing his imagination like this will bring great results.

If he is an open sort of person, try the opposite scenario on him. When you're licking his cock, tell him how much you'd like to have another man filling your pussy while you suck. Indulge in a fantasy of your own about double penetration (being penetrated front and back at the same time) and share it with him. If he is inside you, ask him to imagine if he can feel the other man inside you as well. Double penetration is a common lady's fantasy, and many have been lucky enough to do it in reality. (A practical substitute is to use a dildo or butt plug to fill the unoccupied berth while he fills the other – see below.)

Threesome sex either way is wonderful grist for the fantasy mill, and you will enjoy it even if it goes no further. Remember that in Western culture one man, one woman is the rule, and we find it difficult to expand a relationship to include a third person. My advice on this point is very strong – DON'T TRY A THREE-SIDED RELATIONSHIP. It is inherently unstable and someone will get hurt.

On the other hand, there is everything to recommend using the occasional third person as a sex toy. Everyone I am aware of who has tried it – even if they don't want to do it again – remembers the occasion as hot and exciting. As you would expect, you won't have to ask permission before bringing another woman to your bed. That is one toy your man will have no difficulty playing with. Unfortunately this world is unjust, and you will almost certainly have to tread carefully if you anticipate inviting another man. I suggest you bring the matter up with him in advance and agree that if you ever get an offer of a threesome (of either sex) that meets your conditions, you'll both accept it. Most likely it will never happen, but you can always dream – and fantasizing about missed opportunities will be fun. The conditions are that the third person should not be a close friend, that you both feel comfortable on the night, and that the third partner must do their thing and leave. You don't want anyone to strike up a relationship with either of you, and anyway, you will need time together afterwards to savour the pleasure. I won't talk about the need for safe sex practices when dealing with outsiders – even if they are friends. You should be adult enough to follow these very strictly, so keep some condoms in your bedside drawer – just in case.

If it does happen and you get the chance to take a girl home with you, remember you are the boss. You are lending her a little of your man, so take the lead. It will also make life easier for your man if you tell him what to do. For instance, he might be frightened to go down on her for fear of upsetting you, but if you issue the invitation he can relax and enjoy himself. Likewise, if it is a man you are taking home, he should call the tune – for the same reasons. You will not feel guilty about accommodating a man at both ends if he has asked the man to help fly you to the moon.

Don't be surprised if you do a lot of lovemaking in the hours after the third partner has left. You will be basking in the glow of having been very, very naughty.

There may be active swingers in your town – couples who meet for group sex. These are probably best contacted through the internet. Chat online for a while with both sides of the couple before meeting, and meet at a neutral venue for the first time. Try a bar or restaurant, and if things work out, go with the flow.

Nice alternatives are the swingers' clubs and swingers' holiday resorts that you can find on the internet. These are tremendously variable but look to be fun. They all seem to invite participation, but don't insist on it. If you are lucky enough to live near one, give it a try. Or book a dirty weekend in one of the resorts. It will certainly be something to talk about afterwards. This is one of the things on my personal wish list.

Mirrors, Cameras, Camcorders and Web cams

We all like making love, and we all like watching lovemaking. It adds a certain spice if you can watch his cock burrowing in and out of you. Traditional brothels often mount a large mirror on the ceiling over the bed so lovers can watch themselves. Because of the weight of the glass, ceiling mirrors are a little difficult to install – much harder than hanging a mirror on a wall – and I don't suppose you want your local handyman involved in fitting it. It is also a very clear statement to your mother-in-law when she visits. Instead try fitting sliding mirror doors to your wardrobe and pose your man so you can watch everything happening as you make love. I know you will enjoy it.

Using a camera to record the fun is very much more common now that digital cameras are so widely available. Before that you needed to develop old-fashioned photographs at home, because you did not want the local camera store to spread your intimate pictures over town. Now you can do it yourself with no more equipment than a basic computer. Of course, taking pictures of each other is simple; taking pictures which cover you both is much more difficult. A tripod and remote shutter control are a must.

Camcorders can make for some impressive entertainment. He will definitely want videos of you posing or doing interesting things to yourself, and he will keep them to watch when the real thing is not available. To make a really satisfying video of you both you need a cameraman (or woman). Private blue movie making is available in cities but finding the right person might be difficult.

Arranging a private 'glamour' shoot in a photographic studio is much easier. Photographers do sets for prospective models and often have a complete service involving doing your make-up and showing you how to pose. Others make a business opportunity out of dolling up ordinary folks and turning out glamorous pictures that you just can't believe were possible. Perhaps you think that the camera doesn't lie, but fortunately that is not true. Even an ordinary portrait photographer will present you in a way that will boost your self-esteem. The job of the photographer is to create a series of good quality portraits of a glamorous version of you – clothed, partly clothed or even nude. Your man will appreciate an album like this even if he is the only one that ever sees it. Visit the studio first and make sure you are happy with the photographer and the studio, and that they can do your make-up and posing. Ask to see examples of his (or her) work and if you like what you see, book a session. If you want him there, ask if your man can come too; he will probably enjoy watching you pose and being the centre of attention.

The only thing you need to worry about is that you keep control of the pictures and negatives – for obvious reasons. A reputable studio will have a standard agreement to sign that leaves all the rights and negatives with you.

On the day of the session make sure your hair is in good shape and take make-up, a bikini (preferably a thong one) and nice lingerie with you. Professional models take a little weekend bag for all their things, and they wear loose clothes and no tight underwear or pantyhose because they don't want red marks on their skin. If you are shy about exposing yourself to the camera, go to the studio without a fixed limit in mind of what you are going to show. That way you can pose for pretty pictures of yourself showing a bit of cleavage and work up to whatever you feel comfortable with. Try and let yourself relax and be persuaded to do things that you might not do if you sat and thought about it coldly. You and your man will love the results – a permanent record of a fantasy girl.

Anal Sex

Finally, at the back end of our book (I couldn't resist putting it in such an appropriate place) we come to anal sex. For some people the whole idea is so far beyond the boundaries of what they can accept as normal, that they could never, ever allow a lover to touch them there. On the other hand, even maiden aunts now realize that it is not only limited to the gay community. In fact it is going on everywhere around you and more than half the people on the morning train to work have tried it at some time or other. I don't have any statistics to quote but it seems that most women who have tried it gently with their lovers enjoyed it, and for many of them it has remained a valued part of their sexual menu. Apart from that, you can be sure that your man has certainly thought about trying it with you and if you haven't explored the possibilities already, he will jump at the chance to start.

Anal penetration may also be one of your own fantasies; as I said above, most women have wondered what it would be like to be taken by two men at once. Now is your chance to find out.

119

There are two things you should bear in mind about anal sex. Firstly it's not strange, deviant, degrading, immoral or any other of the negative adjectives you might have heard. Secondly, most women who take the time to learn how to do it successfully find it is amazingly pleasurable.

When your man pats your butt or holds your cheeks in his hands, it feels nice. This is because your anus and the surrounding area is supplied with an amazing network of nerves and playing with your butt wakes them all up to see what is going on. Oh dear, you have already started on the slippery slope, and you didn't even realize it.

If you want to experiment with anal sex, the best way to start is to let your man know that you enjoy the feeling of his fingers in that area. Encourage him if he accidentally strays around there. Or if you are riding him cowgirl position, stop and make a big deal of dolloping some personal lubricant on and around your anus. Then take him out of your pussy and rub him on your anus until he comes (which won't be long). Don't go for penetration at all at this stage; you need to work up to that.

Another way to amuse yourselves is for you to lie with your back to him, on your side with your legs stretched so you are straight, not in a spooning position. Again put plenty of lubrication in the cleft of your ass and holding his cock to keep him under control, let him slide up and down between your cheeks. It will feel fantastic for him – especially when you clench your cheeks on him – and you will enjoy having him brush past your anus as well. Again, don't try to get him inside you at this point, although you may well want to have him pressing against you as he comes. Feeling him spurt in that position is delightful and very exciting.

This sort of play is very stimulating, and having him do exciting things to your anus while you are coming through oral sex adds greatly to the excitement. Eventually you will want to move on and have him inside you, so let's look at the best way to approach that.

Firstly, you need to enlist your man's help. He will be looking forward to the day he can bury himself in your desirable ass, so cooperation won't be a problem, but do make it clear that it is your ass and you are going to be the one in charge. Secondly, you need to reasonably clean. Your rectum is normally empty and a shower with a little more than usual attention to your butt is enough. Finally, agree with him that nothing that's been in your butt is going to be put in your pussy – that's a quick way to an infection. (Going the other direction – pussy to butt – is perfectly safe.)

Your butt is not self-lubricating in the way your pussy is, so a good supply of personal lubricant is vital. Astroglide is the commonest but there are many others. I have heard particularly good things about Eros from Germany. Saliva is just not good enough but baby oil works quite well. Check your man's fingernails for sharp edges, and file them off if you find them.

The great things for beginners to remember are to use twice as much lube as you think is possible, and start small. A good way to start is to get him to rub lube onto your anus while making love doggy style, and then slip the tip of his pinky into you and hold still. Obviously your body can accommodate something this small very easily, but you may experience a little resistance because it is the first time. Try breathing deeply and press out against his finger as if you were having a bowel movement. This will allow him to slip in easily and providing you have enough lubricant, you will not experience a 'burning' sensation. Warn him that you will pull his finger out when you've had enough, and in the meantime he is not to move in and out. Once you have relaxed around his finger, you will find that the feeling of being 'full' adds to the sensations of lovemaking in your pussy. You will enjoy your orgasm, but may feel that you need to take him out immediately afterwards. This is a fairly common reaction immediately after orgasm, so don't be surprised.

Discuss what happened once you cool down and let him know if he needs to do anything different. If it felt wonderful, share the experience with him. If it just felt uncomfortable, you were doing it incorrectly – not enough lube, no relaxing etc. – and you will do better next time.

A possible next step is to buy a butt plug or two. A butt plug is a teardrop-shaped blob of plastic gel mounted by a narrower shaft onto a flared base. The pointed end lets it slip easily into a well-lubed ass; the narrow shaft allows your muscles to close again behind the larger diameter teardrop, and the flared base makes sure it doesn't slip in too far and get lost. Buy a slim one for your early attempts. You can get him to slide it into you during foreplay, or use it during lovemaking. Both are good and you will enjoy the feeling of being filled from both sides as you make love. Don't be surprised if you squeeze it out as you come; that is just your contractions treating it like squeezing an orange pip.

A slim butt plug is still much smaller than a cock, so you need to buy something a bit bigger to get used to relaxing around him. Try a Tristan plug. Visit www.vixencreations.com if you can't find one in your local shop. This plug was designed by the famous anal expert, Tristan Taormino. (Can you imagine that for a career? Being an expert in anal sex – what does she put down on her IRS return?) The Tristan plug is designed to be used by someone who is already used to relaxing around a smaller plug, but given enough lube and enough time, you should have no trouble enjoying it. Its neck is relatively long which means that once it is inside you, the head is past the rings of muscle around your anus and the plug is unlikely to slip out no matter what other lovemaking you do.

Finally you should feel confident enough to accept your lover. First relax yourself by having an orgasm or two, and by using your largest butt plug. Chose a position. If your hips are around the same width as your man's and making love in the 'spoon' position is easy for you, this is probably the best one to start with. Doggy style is an alternative, or even on your back with your knees pulled up towards your shoulders. Whichever you choose, cover his cock with lots of lube, pull out the butt plug and guide him in, keeping your hand on him to control the depth and speed of penetration. Once he is in, have him lie still for a while until you are relaxed around him. Experiment with a little movement; if you are not comfortable, have him pull out and add some more lube to both of you before trying again. Don't worry if movement is uncomfortable on this first occasion. Celebrate progress by giving yourself an orgasm and then pull him out and bring him off by hand. Next time will be even better. Many women who never orgasm unassisted during conventional sex have the most fantastic orgasms during anal sex, and that is where you are headed.

This is what Nymuweah (another expert) has to say about being penetrated by her lover. "I love the sensation of feeling my ass slowly being filled by his cock. I feel like I'm swallowing him. I really like to control the pace by being the one to slowly push back on him at the pace I'm ready to take him. And once he's fully inside, there is nothing else like that! One of the most exquisite sensations for me of anal sex is when he pulls out and then slides back in the first time. The in-stroke is absolutely amazingly pleasurable for me. I can't help but moan and push back towards him. I love it." Sounds good to me too.

Working on the principle that what's sauce for the goose is also sauce for the gander, you may find that he fantasizes about being penetrated by you. This idea can be a little touchy as some men seem to think that any feeling in that direction is an admission of latent homosexuality. That might sound stupid to you – it sounds absolutely crazy to me – but there it is. Some men are completely uptight about their virgin butt, and if you have a man like this he won't hesitate to let you know if your fingers wander in that direction. On the other hand, if he seems open to new things, approach him in the same way that I recommended he approach you (remember the postilion technique I told you about in the chapter on oral sex).

If he is enjoying you massaging his prostate with a well-lubricated finger or butt plug, you're in luck. Rush to the www.vixencreations.com website and order a Nexus double dildo and a harness to hold it in place. This is an absolutely magic piece of equipment. It consists of a dildo that reaches up inside you, wraps around between your lips and rests against your clit. And best of all, it has an elegant cock projecting out in front of you at just the right angle. Use the harness to hold it in place and you have a cock to pleasure the neighbourhood with.

Another amazing alternative is the Feeldoe. Designed by women for women, it also has a bulb that fits inside you at just the right angle to leave a useful cock sticking out in front.

Buy either of them together on the internet and tell him you want one to use on the next girlfriend he brings home. Warn him that he can't quickly find a girl for you to practice on, you're going to use it on him. He'll be opening the package with trembling hands when it finally arrives. You never know, he might find a girl for you to try, but I'm sure it won't be until he's tried it himself.

And so! On to the Final Frontier!

What is the final frontier when you're fantasizing? Of course, there isn't one. There are no limits to what you can dream about, and often the excitement of dreaming exceeds reality. So keep on doing a little of this and that, and dreaming a lot about everything else. It is a guaranteed good ride.

Oh, and as I sign off at the end of our romp through various aspects of sexual attraction and subjugating your man with ecstasy, how are you feeling? Did you learn anything? Are you seeing things a little differently? Are you itching to get on and try to make your love life even better? I hope so; the world needs more lovers and you must do your bit. It's your duty and it's fun!

Extras

While researching material for this book I found I was accumulating a great many intriguing quotations from famous people about lovers and sex. I used some of them but could not bear to just throw the rest away. So here they are, the wisdom of the ancients about our most ancient pastime (plus a few oddities like the one from Emperor Hirohito that I just could not resist).

Love is the answer, but while you're waiting for the answer, sex raises some pretty interesting questions. **Woody Allen**

Jacqueline George

The prison psychiatrist asked me if I thought sex was dirty. I told him only when it's done right. Woody Allen

Sex without love is an empty experience, but as empty experiences go it's one of the best. Woody Allen

All women become like their mothers. That is their tragedy. No man does. That's his. Oscar Wilde *The Importance of Being Earnest*

Life is too important to be taken seriously. Oscar Wilde

Pussy rules the world. Madonna

Do not go baggy when dressing, because this style only adds weight to your figure. Balance out your outfit by wearing a full skirt and then a fitted shirt or a flowing blouse with fitted pants. Darla Ott - Springfield - USA

It is one of the superstitions of the human mind to have imagined that virginity could be a virtue. Voltaire

My girlfriend always laughs during sex – no matter what she's reading. Steve Jobs

People make love for so many crazy reasons – why shouldn't money be one of them? Ben Gazzara

How to make Wild, Passionate Love to your Man

Love built on beauty, soon as beauty, dies.
John Donne 1572-1631: *The Anagram* (c1595)

Licence my roving hands, and let them go,
Behind, before, above, between, below.
O my America, my new found land,
My kingdom, safeliest when with one man manned.
John Donne 1572-1631: *To His Mistress Going to Bed* (c1595)

'Goodness, what beautiful diamonds!'
'Goodness had nothing to do with it.'

Mae West 1892-1980: *Night After Night* (1932 film)

Personally I know nothing about sex because I've always been
married.

Zsa Zsa Gabor

When I hear his steps outside my door I lie down on my bed,
close my eyes, open my legs, and think of England.

Lady Hillingdon 1857-1940: diary, 1912)

'Tisn't beauty, so to speak, nor good talk necessarily. It's just It.
Some women'll stay in a man's memory if they once walked down a
street.

Rudyard Kipling 1865-1936: *Traffics and Discoveries* (1904)

The Duke returned from the wars today and did pleasure me in
his top-boots.

Sarah, Duchess of Marlborough 1660-1744

Is that a gun in your pocket, or are you just glad to see me?

Mae West

There is no excellent beauty that hath not some strangeness in the proportion.

Francis Bacon 1561-1626: *Essays* (1625) *Of Beauty*

She walks in beauty, like the night
Of cloudless climes and starry skies;
And all that's best of dark and bright
Meet in her aspect and her eyes.
Lord Byron 1788-1824: *She Walks in Beauty* (1815)

Near this spot are deposited the remains of one who possessed beauty without vanity, strength without insolence, courage without ferocity, and all the virtues of Man, without his vices.

Lord Byron 1788-1824: *Inscription on the Monument of a Newfoundland Dog* (1808)

Beauty is no quality in things themselves. It exists merely in the mind which contemplates them.

David Hume 1711-76: *Of the Standard of Taste* (1757)

We are all in the gutter, but some of us are looking at the stars.

Oscar Wilde *Lady Windermere's Fan* (1892)

There is no such thing as a moral or an immoral book. Books are well written, or badly written.

Oscar Wilde 1854-1900: *The Picture of Dorian Gray* (1891)

Love is two minutes fifty-two seconds of squishing noises.
Johnny Rotten 1957- *Daily Mirror*, 1983

Tracy: Let's fool around. Let's do it some strange way that you've always wanted to, but nobody would do with you.

Manhattan, the movie

Any woman could act like a lady, and this behaviour was interpreted as being submissive, demure, inhibited. Being a lady in the Western world was like foot binding in China.

Victoria Billings

A kiss is a lovely trick designed by nature to stop speech when words become superfluous.

Ingrid Bergman

Gentlemen prefer blondes. Anita Loos

The hair is the richest ornament of women. Martin Luther

Being a woman is a terribly difficult task since it consists principally in dealing with men. Joseph Conrad

Never eat anything at one sitting that you can't lift. Miss Piggy

Brevity is the soul of lingerie. Dorothy Parker

If you want to know what God thinks of money, just look at the people he gave it to.

Dorothy Parker

You'd be surprised how much it costs to look this cheap.

Dolly Parton

Trust me, Paulette, you have all the equipment. You just need to read the manual.

Elle Woods in *Legally Blonde*

If men can run the world, why can't they stop wearing neckties? How intelligent is it to start the day by tying a little noose around your neck?

Linda Ellerbee

I am a marvellous housekeeper. Every time I leave a man I keep his house.

Zsa Zsa Gabor

I never married because there was no need. I have three pets at home which answer the same purpose as a husband. I have a dog which

growls every morning, a parrot which swears all afternoon and a cat that comes home late at night.

Marie Corelli

There are a number of mechanical devices that increase sexual arousal, particularly in women. Chief amongst these is the Mercedes Benz 380L convertible.

PJ O'Rourke

The big difference between sex for money and sex for free is that sex for money costs less. Brendan Francis

A nymphomaniac is a woman as obsessed with sex as the average man.

Mignon McLaughlin

I believe that sex is a beautiful thing between two people. Between five, it's fantastic.

Woody Allen on Sex

If there is reincarnation, I'd like to come back as Pamela Anderson's fingertips.

Woody Allen on Sex

I'm such a good lover because I practice a lot on my own.

Woody Allen on Sex

My love life is terrible. The last time I was inside a woman was when I visited the Statue of Liberty.

Jacqueline George

Woody Allen on Sex

Everything has beauty, but not everyone sees it. Confucius

Scientists have discovered a food that diminishes a woman's sex drive by 90%. It's called a wedding cake. Anon.

There's no such thing as a free lunch. Milton Friedman

A man is only as old as the woman he feels. Groucho Marx

I chased a woman for almost two years only to discover her tastes were exactly like mine – we were both crazy about girls.

Groucho Marx

Nancy Astor (to Winston Churchill): *If I were your wife I would put poison in your coffee!*

Churchill: *And if I were your husband I would drink it.*

Bessie Braddock (to Winston Churchill): *Winston, you're drunk.*

Churchill: *Bessie, you're ugly. But tomorrow I shall be sober.*

Whatever women do they must do twice as well as men to be thought half as good. Luckily, this is not difficult.

Charlotte Whitton

How to make Wild, Passionate Love to your Man

The war has developed not necessarily to Japan's advantage.
Emperor Hirohito, announcing Japan's surrender after atom bombs
destroyed Hiroshima and Nagasaki

*Biologically speaking, if something bites you, it is more likely to
be female.* Desmond Morris

*When I'm good, I'm very, very good, but when I'm bad, I'm
better.*

Mae West

*I once had a rose named after me and I was very flattered. But I
was not pleased to read the description in the catalogue: no good in a
bed, but fine up against a wall.*

Eleanor Roosevelt

I had the radio on. Marilyn Monroe, asked if she really had
nothing on in a calendar photograph

Chanel No. 5. Marilyn Monroe, asked what she wore in bed

*Clinton lied. A man might forget where he parks or where he
lives, but he never forgets oral sex, no matter how bad it is.*

Barbara Bush

*According to a new survey, women say they feel more
comfortable undressing in front of men than they do undressing in
front of other women. They say that women are too judgmental,
where, of course, men are just grateful.*

Jacqueline George

Robert De Niro

*There's very little advice in men's magazines, because men think,
I know what I'm doing. Just show me somebody naked.*

Jerry Seinfield

*See, the problem is that God gives men a brain and a penis, and
only enough blood to run one at a time.* Robin Williams

*The good people sleep much better at night than the bad people.
Of course, the bad people enjoy the waking hours much more.*
Woody Allen

*Aphrodite is only more attractive when united with Bacchus; their
pleasures are sweeter for being mixed together.*

Lucian of Samosata

Beauty comes in all sizes — not just size 5.

Roseanne

*God gave women intuition and femininity. Used properly, the
combination easily jumbles the brain of any man I've ever met.*
Farrah Fawcett

When women go wrong, men go right after them.

Mae West

How to make Wild, Passionate Love to your Man

Being a sex symbol has to do with an attitude, not looks. Most men think it's looks, most women know otherwise.

Kathleen Turner

A woman who has the divine gift of lechery and loves her partner will masturbate him well – subtly, unhurriedly and mercilessly.

Dr Alex Comfort

We desire nothing so much as what we ought not to have.

Publilius Syrus ~100 BC,

The definition of a beautiful woman is one who loves me.

Sloan Wilson

A man is already halfway in love with any woman who listens to him.

Brendan Francis

You don't love a woman because she is beautiful, but she is beautiful because you love her. Anon.

We are all born for love. It is the principle of existence, and its only end.

Benjamin Disraeli

There are times not to flirt. When you're sick. When you're with children. When you're on the witness stand.

Jacqueline George

Joyce Jillson

Girls are always running through my mind. They don't dare walk.

Andy Gibb

Good girls go to heaven, bad girls go everywhere.

Helen Gurley Brown

People are more violently opposed to fur than leather because it's safer to harass rich women than motorcycle gangs. Anon.

When the candles are out all women are fair.

Plutarch (46 – 120 AD)

Women who seek to be equal with men lack ambition.

Timothy Leary

Women with pasts interest men... they hope history will repeat itself.

Mae West

If women didn't exist, all the money in the world would have no meaning.

Aristotle Onassis

American women expect to find in their husbands a perfection that English women only hope to find in their butlers.

How to make Wild, Passionate Love to your Man

Somerset Maugham

I married beneath me – all women do. Nancy Astor

I love the women's movement... especially when I'm walking behind it.

Rush Limbaugh

GARTHER, n. An elastic band intended to keep a woman from coming out of her stockings and desolating the country.

Ambrose Bierce *The Devil's Dictionary*

I have too many fantasies to be a housewife. I guess I am a fantasy. Marilyn Monroe

If a thing is worth doing, it is worth doing slowly... very slowly.

Gypsy Rose Lee

My mother was like a sister to me, only we didn't have sex quite so often.

Emo Philips

It is impossible to obtain a conviction for sodomy from an English jury. Half of them don't believe that it can physically be done, and the other half are doing it.

Winston Churchill

Jacqueline George

When the authorities warn you of the dangers of having sex, there is an important lesson to be learnt. Do not have sex with the authorities.

Homer Simpson

If you've got them by the balls, their hearts and minds will follow.

John Wayne

You know how a woman gets a man excited? She shows up. That's it; we're guys, we're easy.

Harrison Ford in *Six Days Seven Nights*

She must always lay stress on closing and constricting the Yoni (the vagina) until it holds the Lingam (the penis) as with a fist, opening and shutting at her pleasure, and finally acting as the hand of the Gopala-girl who milks the cow. This can be learned only by long practice, and especially by throwing the will into the part affected. Her husband will then value her above all women, nor would he exchange her for the most beautiful queen in the Three Worlds... Karma Sutra

We cannot, by an effort of the will, either command or restrain the erection of the penis; and yet it is evidently owing to the mind; for sudden fear, or anything which fixes our attention strongly and all at

137

How to make Wild, Passionate Love to your Man

once, makes this member quickly subside, though it were ever so fully erected.

Robert Whytt 1751

A life is more valuable than a penis.

Lisa Kemler, Lorena Bobbitt's attorney, arguing for her client who severed her husband's penis, which was later reattached.

"Do you believe in love at first sight, or should I walk by again?"
Anon

The anatomy of the clitoris was described in 1559 by Renaldus Columbus of Padua, who claimed that previous anatomists had overlooked the very existence of 'so pretty a thing'. Leslet A Hall

Wouldn't be any fun if they just fell over with their legs in the air.
Cocktail, the movie

Sex on the television can't hurt you unless you fall off.
skoper@world.std.com

Why is it that when they show a computer ad they show computers and when they show a car ad they show cars but when they show a condom ad they show people playing tennis?
steven.sullivan@office.wang.com

Men want the same things from a relationship as women.....only
MORE SEX! T-Rex

Men never do evil so completely and cheerfully as when they do it from religious conviction.

Blaise Pascal

Baroque -- not having enough Monet... zinger

Behind every great woman -- is her butt. zinger

I don't understand girls. They want something but they don't tell you what. You're supposed to guess! Girls scare me, they're different than us! The Family Guy, Stewie

When a lady is left wide awake, a gentleman has not done his duty.

Judging Amy

Whether they give or refuse, it delights women just the same to have been asked. Ovid

Once, during prohibition, I was forced to live for days on nothing but food and water. W.C. Fields

First they came for the Communists, but I didn't speak up because I wasn't a Communist. Then they came for the Jews, but I didn't speak up because I wasn't a Jew... Then they came for me, and I said, "Wait! You forgot about the gays! And I know where they're hiding!"

Angus Johnston

How to make Wild, Passionate Love to your Man

People only say I remind them of Liz Taylor because I'm not skinny.

Christina Ricci

Elizabeth Taylor is pre-feminist woman. This is the source of her continuing greatness and relevance. She wields the sexual power that feminism cannot explain and has tried to destroy. Camille Paglia

Feminist anti-porn discourse virtually always ignores the gigantic gay male porn industry, since any mention of the latter would bring crashing to the ground the absurd argument that pornography is by definition subordination of women... Far from poisoning the mind, pornography shows the deepest truth about sexuality, stripped of romantic veneer... What feminists denounce as woman's humiliating total accessibility in porn is actually her elevation to high priestess of a pagan paradise garden, where the body has become a bountiful fruit tree where growth and harvest are simultaneous.

Camille Paglia

It is woman's destiny to rule men. Not to serve them, flatter them, or hang on them for guidance. Nor to insult them, demean them, or stereotype them as oppressors. ...It is not male hatred of women but male fear of women that is the great universal. Camille Paglia

Let's get rid of Infirmary Feminism, with its bedlam of bellyachers, anorexics, bulimics, depressives, rape victims, and incest survivors. Feminism has become a catch-all vegetable drawer where bunches of clingy sob sisters can store their mouldy neuroses.
Camille Paglia

Sex is a far darker power than feminism has admitted. Sex is the point of contact between man and nature, where morality and good intentions fall to primitive urges. Camille Paglia

Men have been trained and conditioned by women, not unlike the way Pavlov conditioned his dogs, into becoming their slaves. As compensation for their labours men are given periodic use of a woman's vagina. Esther Vilar

The rarest thing in the world is a woman who is pleased with photographs of herself.

Elizabeth Metcalf

The most popular image of the female despite the exigencies of the clothing trade is all boobs and buttocks, a hallucinating sequence of parabolae and bulges.

Germaine Greer

The essence of life is the smile of round female bottoms. Guy de Maupassant

Women dress alike all over the world: they dress to be annoying to other women.

Isa Schiaparelli

She wore a short skirt and a tight sweater and her figure described a set of parabolas that could cause cardiac arrest in a yak.

Woody Allen, *Getting Even*

How to make Wild, Passionate Love to your Man

Life without sex might be safer but it would be unbearably dull. It is the sex instinct which makes women seem beautiful, which they are once in a blue moon, and men seem wise and brave, which they never are at all. Throttle it, denaturalize it, take it away, and human existence would be reduced to the prosaic, laborious, boresome, imbecile level of life in an anthill. Henry Louis Mencken

Men wake up aroused in the morning. We can't help it. We just wake up and we want you. And the women are thinking, "How can he want me the way I look in the morning?" It's because we can't see you. We have no blood anywhere near our optic nerve. Andy Rooney

Why should we take advice on sex from the pope? If he knows anything about it, he shouldn't!

George Bernard Shaw

Conservatives say teaching sex education in the public schools will promote promiscuity. With our education system? If we promote promiscuity the same way we promote math or science, they've got nothing to worry about.

Beverly Mickins

It is not economical to go to bed early to save the candles if the result is twins. Chinese Proverb

Obscenity is whatever gives the Judge an erection. Anon

When a man goes on a date he wonders if he is going to get lucky. A woman already knows.

Jacqueline George

Frederike Ryder

I *regret to say that we of the FBI are powerless to act in cases of oral-genital intimacy, unless it has in some way obstructed interstate commerce.*

J. Edgar Hoover

Who would give a law to lovers? Love is unto itself a higher law.

Boethius, *The Consolation of Philosophy*, A.D. 524

Some women can't say the word lesbian even when their mouth is full of one.

Kate Clinton

There's a difference between beauty and charm. A beautiful woman is one I notice. A charming woman is one who notices me.

John Erskine

A dress makes no sense unless it inspires men to want to take it off you.

Françoise Sagan

Remember that always dressing in understated good taste is the same as playing dead.

Susan Catherine

A skirt is no obstacle to extemporaneous sex, but it is physically

How to make Wild, Passionate Love to your Man

impossible to make love to a girl while she is wearing trousers.
Helen Lawrenson

Those hot pants of hers were so damned tight, I could hardly breathe.

Benny Hill

A woman reading Playboy feels a little like a Jew reading a Nazi manual.

Gloria Steinem

What they love to yield they would often rather have stolen. Rough seduction delights them, the boldness of near rape is a compliment.

Ovid, *The Art of Love*

Women and cats will do as they please, and men and dogs should relax and get used to the idea.

Robert A Heinlein

Discontented women dream of being rescued by Prince Charming. Discontented men dream of finding a horny blond in the back seat of a taxi.

Mason Cooley

The difference between pornography and erotica is lighting.
Gloria Leonard

Jacqueline George

When I want to read a good book, I write one.

Benjamin Disraeli

You're the one I want to forever please, lick you, suck you, taste you and tease.

Rhonda *Forever Kind of Ecstasy*

If a man is talking in the forest, and there is no woman there to hear him, is he still wrong?

Jenny Weber

The great question – which I have not been able to answer – is, 'What does a woman want?'

Sigmund Freud

They were doing a full back shot of me in a swimsuit and I thought, Oh my God, I have to be so brave. See, every woman hates herself from behind.

Cindy Crawford

Sally wears a size two dress, and going to bed with her would be like going to bed with a bicycle.

Erica Jong *Any Woman's Blues*

"What do you take me for, an idiot?"

General Charles de Gaulle (1890-1970), when a journalist asked him if he was happy

How to make Wild, Passionate Love to your Man

One of the symptoms of an approaching nervous breakdown is the belief that one's work is terribly important.

Bertrand Russell

He who hesitates is a damned fool. Mae West

Manuscript: something submitted in haste and returned at leisure.

Oliver Herford

When choosing between two evils, I always like to try the one I've never tried before.

Mae West

I don't want to achieve immortality through my work; I want to achieve immortality through not dying.

Woody Allen

Some editors are failed writers, but so are most writers.

T. S. Eliot (1888-1965)

Heav'n hath no rage like love to hatred turn'd, Nor Hell a fury like a woman scorn'd.

William Congreve

We don't like their sound, and guitar music is on the way out.

Jacqueline George

Decca Recording Co. rejecting the Beatles, 1962

Pray, v.: To ask that the laws of the universe be annulled on behalf of a single petitioner, confessedly unworthy. Ambrose Bierce

I choose a block of marble and chop off whatever I don't need. Francois-Auguste Rodin (1840-1917), when asked how he managed to make his remarkable statues

Happiness is watching the TV at your girlfriend's house during a power failure.

Bob Hope

I love the idea of there being two sexes, don't you?

James Thurber

Believe me, my young friend, there is nothing – absolutely nothing – half so much worth doing as simply messing about in women.

with apologies to Kenneth Grahame

'How about it, Sis –I mean, like can you come on top?'

'You silly-billy,' she chided 'I can come on card tricks!'

Terry Southern *Blue Movie*

Other titles by Jacqueline George

The Prince and the Nun

Foreign Affairs

Her Master's Voice

Light o'Love

Falling into Queensland

The Accidental Spy

Where Gold Lies

www.jacquelinegeorgewriter.com

www.ingramcontent.com/pod-product-compliance
Lightning Source LLC
Chambersburg PA
CBHW060521290526
45791CB00001B/480

9 781495 436383